Nursing Homes,

Heaven Or Hell?

A true story of what Nursing Home Living could be like for you or a loved one.

Author

Joyce M. Poxon

Retired Activity Director

This book is a work of non-fiction. Names and places have been changed to protect the privacy of all individuals. The events and situations are true.

ISBN: 1-4107-7199-7 (e-book)
ISBN: 1-4107-7200-4 (Paperback)

Library of Congress Control Number: 2003094927

This book is printed on acid free paper.

Printed in the United States of America
Bloomington, IN

1stBooks - rev. 12/10/03

INDEX

CHAPTER

ACKNOWLEDGEMENTS

I would like to acknowledge the following individuals who helped me achieve success throughout the years.

Listed in alphabetical order

Departmental Assistants

Marilyn Antinio, Anthony Barrigan,
Geneva Bennett, Darci Browning, Marvin Cobbs,
Linda Dubose, Anna Elerbee, Lee Erwin,
Joy Freeman, Tanaya Gainey, Lidia Gonka,
Nicole Hess, Verla Hill, Nicole Jones,
Phyllis Jones, Navy Loshnjian, Thelma Moore,
Shannon Morgan, Karen Newman, Merley Risker,
Barry Rubin, Rhonda Williams

Outstanding Volunteers

Cathy Davis,
Jill Fogerty,
Patty Meyer,
Carmen Santos

ACKNOWLEDGEMENTS CONTINUED

Outstanding Adult Education Teachers

Doctor Tom Craven
and Lois Schenker

And

My husband, John
who shared the good times
and helped me through the bad times of my career.

Their support, devotion and hard work
made my success possible.

Thank you all.
I could not have done it without you.

A special thanks to Doctor Tom Craven for his encouragement,
persistence and assistance in completing this book.

PREFACE

Books have been written about nursing homes from the prospective of individuals who have never worked in one.

However, my book covers the story as seen from the inside, what goes on behind the scenes, the good and the bad.

I hope you will find my experiences interesting and enjoyable and my point of view enlightening as it is about the enjoyable times, the rewards and blessings I received by making a difference as well as heartaches and tribulations I experienced that were all a part of working in the field.

So many indviduals who have ever worked in an activity department for a nursing home will undoubtedly relate to what I have written for it is a position that takes a truly dedicated and high energy level individual to perform the duties required.

I was once told, "Only good activity directors suffer burn out." Although that is true, it doesn't have to be that way. Dedicated individuals should not be punished for doing a good job.

CHAPTER 1

INTRODUCTION

"Nursing Homes, Heaven or Hell?" is nonfiction based on what I was personally involved in or witnessed during my many years of employment in nursing homes and what compelled me to write about my experiences.

Although many of my nursing home experiences were gratifying, heart warming and humorous, most were very stressful and some so horrifying they forever changed the life of many individuals, including my own.

Portions of this book are dedicated to a behind the scenes view of nursing homes regarding the existing conditions and problems with everyone who is involved in their operation including government and state regulators, owners, administrators, staff, to the residents themselves.

Included are guidelines on how to select a good nursing home with a list of do's and don'ts for those who have already selected a facility.

I do not claim to have full knowledge of the total operation of nursing homes. But, having spent a good part of my time in them, has given me first hand knowledge on how they are run, the positives, the negatives and the State mandated requirements and I know what should be considered before selecting any health care facility.

Also included are my experiences of why and how I got into the field of activities beginning with my volunteer services then employment in independent living facilities and several nursing homes.

I have been verbally recognized by the State of California as being one of the best in the field. I have set up departments for other facilities and trained their staff. In addition, I have composed, designed and have copy righted the forms and activity calendar that several facilities are using.

I am proud of my accomplishments. However the thing I am most proud of is that I have made a difference in the life of so many and for that I am grateful for I have been richly blessed.

Doctors and nurses can help heal the body, but not the heart and mind. Resident activities are intricate parts in the total healing process, as one's body will not mend if the heart and mind are allowed to remain ill by the loss of enjoyment, mental and physical stimulation, self esteem and pride in accomplishment.

Therefore, when selecting a nursing home, it is extremely important that the facility provide a good activity department with quality activity programs that are designed to meet the needs of all of its residents regardless of age or mental or physical abilities.

If anyone should ask me why I stayed in the field of such a stressful position as an Activity Director there could only be one answer. The answer would be, God gave me the burden, stamina, dedication and knowledge of how to help those who needed someone to care and blessed me in doing so.

So many of my experiences working with the elderly and handicapped were so gratifying and rewarding I received much more then I ever gave.

CHAPTER 2

VOLUNTEERING

My first introduction to activity work started when I volunteered for a local nursing home in Indiana. I must confess that my reason for volunteering in the beginning was strictly selfish and personal. My three children were almost grown; I was a single parent going through a troublesome time and felt I needed something meaningful in my life that would help me regain my self esteem.

My sister-in-law asked me if I had ever thought of volunteering in a nursing home. I hadn't thought of it because I hadn't been in a nursing home and didn't even know they used volunteers. The only volunteer work I had done in the past involved my children's school and sport activities. One other time I worked for a political party handing out literature prior to an election.

After giving it some thought I decided to give it a try and I phoned the administrator of a local nursing home.

I informed her of my need and asked if she had a lady who didn't have anyone and could use a visitor. She told me she had the perfect lady for me. She told me the lady's name was Anna. She had Parkinson's disease but was very alert. So I made arrangements to come by the next evening to meet her.

When I arrived the administrator took me in to meet Anna. I didn't stay long the first visit, but made arrangements to come by once a week beginning the following week.

Not knowing Anna or what we would talk about when I went back the next week I took my family photo album to share information about my family as I pointed out their pictures. The visit went smoothly and when I left I felt more confident about my pending friendship with Anna and in the following days I found myself anxiously awaiting my next visit.

When I arrived the following week, Anna greeted me with a smile and she told me about her life. She was a widow, only sixty four years old. She had no children of her own, but had an adopted son whom she hadn't seen in three years. She had lived alone and because of the unsteadiness caused by her disease she had fallen and was sent to the hospital by a neighbor. The hospital called her son who was an attorney in the next town. While she was in the hospital he sold her home, all of her belongings and placed her in the nursing home and had only been to see her one time to finalize some of her financial matters.

My heart ached to see the pain she was going through and I couldn't understand how her son could turn his back on the one who had given him a home, raised him with a mother's love and sacrificed to see that he got a good education.

When it was time for me to leave I left with a real burden for Anna as well as the other residents I saw sitting in front of the television looking so alone and sad. I realized how lucky I was to have a home and family who cared about me.

Within a few days I convinced a couple of my friends to go with me one night a week to visit two more ladies. Sometimes we would visit with all three in the home and other times we would take them out for pie and coffee or an ice cream cone and on several occasions I took Anna to my home for dinner with my family.

Realizing the residents didn't have much to do for recreation I called the administrator and got permission to bring in some programs. The first people I called were my brother and his wife as he played a guitar and he and his wife sang as a duet in their church. They agreed to come and they brought a puppet show. The following week they convinced their church to hold religious services once a week.

I contacted the schools and asked if they had bands and or choirs that could volunteer to perform and they all agreed to come once a month. Before I knew it I had several programs scheduled. The residents really enjoyed themselves immensely.

Then I contacted local businesses and asked for donations for Christmas gifts for the nursing home residents. Everyone was willing to help. After I retrieved all of the donated items I picked up Anna and took her to my house to help me gift wrap everything. Of course she was unable to assist much with the wrapping except to hold her finger on the ribbon while I tied the knots and bows, but she sure enjoyed being a part of it.

At the time I didn't know anything about what was required for providing activities in a nursing home and I worked strictly with the administrator who never said anything about an activity department. I had never heard of certification, Title 22 or State surveys. I only knew those people needed more in their lives than they were getting. I decided I would do what I could to make their life a little more enjoyable.

The time I spent with Anna and the others in the programs I had scheduled gave me so much more than I gave that I left every time feeling refreshed and blessed. The love, appreciation and acknowledgement I received for my efforts made me feel good about myself and helped me regain my self esteem and for the first time in a long time I liked me.

I continued visiting Anna until I moved to California and remarried. Leaving her was hard on both of us, but she understood and gave her blessings. I promised I would keep in touch with her through the mail and phone calls and that I would visit her on return trips back to visit family. I kept in contact with her and although she couldn't write, the administrator kept me informed.

After a few months I returned to Indiana to spend Christmas with my family and I went to visit Anna. When I arrived at the nursing home I was told she had suffered a stroke and was in the hospital. So I went to see her. When I arrived the nurse told me

7

Anna was in a coma and things didn't look good as they were unable to get any response from her and felt it was just a matter of time. I explained who I was and asked if I could go in to see her. The nurse gave me permission but told me not to expect much as she probably wouldn't even know I was there.

I walked to her bedside, touched her arm and called out her name but there was no response. I again called her name and asked her to open her eyes, but still no response. The third time I said, "Anna, this is Joyce, I've come for a visit, please open your eyes and talk to me." With that she opened her eyes, smiled and said, "I knew you would come." Within minutes she asked me to raise the head of her bed so we could visit.

When the nurse came in she was shocked and stated "I can't believe it. We have tried everything to get her to respond with no results. you come in and within minutes she is sitting up talking and laughing."

When it was time for visiting hours to end for the day I promised Anna I would return to see her the next day and I left the hospital feeling that God had surely blessed me with a miracle. If I hadn't known it before I knew then that love and kindness can cross all barriers.

The following day I went to see Anna and was told she would be going home later in the day as she was doing fine. The third time I visited Anna was in the nursing home and we again had a wonderful time visiting and reminiscing. Since I would be leaving for California the next day I had to say good-bye but promised I would be back to see her on my next trip back to Indiana.

However, that was the last time I ever saw my friend Anna as she passed away a few months later in her sleep. Although it was painful to lose her I am so thankful that I was able to spend some quality time with her before she passed and I know her last few months were happier because of me.

With the experiences I had with my friend and the way my volunteer work in the nursing home had all come together I felt that this must surely be my purpose in life. I felt I had been given a gift to work with the sick and elderly. I was not a nurse to help heal their bodies, but a tool that God could use to help heal their hearts and bring a smile to their faces at a time when they have so little to smile about.

Even though at the time I was volunteering I believed God had blessed me with a gift to work in Activities, I had no idea that it would end up being my career for twenty two years. I truly think this was in the master plan all along.

CHAPTER 3

PICKING UP WHERE I LEFT OFF

After our relocation to California my volunteer work was put on the back burner while we were adjusting to our new lives and new jobs. We bought a mobile home in a senior park and it was then that I began my volunteer work again.

I was asked to be the president of the Bonita Paradise community Recreation Association and I accepted. Though I had no connections in California I did have experience on how to solicit free services because I had done that in Indiana.

I began scheduling events, started fund raisers to pay for entertainment and passed out flyers to promote the new program. With the first event the attendance increased from what it was in the past. In a few months the attendance went from twenty-five to eighty-five and then one hundred.

In less than two years my company went out of business and I was in the job market. Some of the residents of our community suggested that I try to get a job in Nursing Home activities where my talents lay and get paid for the work I had been doing for free.

I began scanning the papers to see if anything was available in activities. There were several ads, but most of them were written in a manner I didn't understand at the time such as, "local SNF seeking experienced, certified activity director with full knowledge of Title 22."

I called on two or three of them and, for reasons that I didn't understand at the time, they didn't even want to talk to me if I didn't know what these terms meant. They stated if I was unfamiliar with the requirements than I was not qualified for the position they offered.

So I decided to try again, but this time I would ask to speak with the activity department and ask them what the terms meant and where I could go to be certified. However, when I called, the classes were not to begin for a few months and I needed employment immediately.

Then I spotted an ad that didn't require certification. It was an independent living apartment complex that housed between eight hundred and a thousand residents. Although it wasn't a nursing home it was working in activities and with seniors.

I called and told the administrator I had volunteer experience and could supply her with letters of reference. She had me come in for an interview and took me across the street to the recreation center where they held all of their activities, gave me a tour of the complex and hired me that same day.

CHAPTER 4

WORKING IN INDEPENDENT LIVING

I started my first day by attending a meeting with their resident association where the administrator introduced me as their new activity director. Then I met separately with their ladies and men's clubs.

I prepared a questionnaire asking what type of activities they would like to see happen in their community and the response was great. I didn't have a budget so I started fund raisers. I scheduled entertainers, parties, dances and sold tickets to cover the cost. I guess they were hungry for good programs because I had a large audience the first time and each time the attendance increased to the point I would have to stop selling tickets in advance to stay within the allowed occupancy limit of the hall and I had resident volunteers coming out of the wood work to help where ever I needed them. Can you imagine that? A previous volunteer now had volunteers.

We had weekly entertainment that included some local television personalities who were also performers, special events of summer fairs that were broadcast on a local radio station and an authentic English Tea where the code of dress was formal from head to toe. We even had a door man dressed in a tuxedo, top hat and cane who announced each guest as they entered the room giving them royalty titles such as, queen, king, prince, princes, etc. and I had authentic English food catered.

All of the parties, special events and fund raisers were huge successes. With the extra cash brought in I was able to replace some needed equipment, some small appliances for the kitchen and a sixty-one inch colored television.

For the next two years things were going well. It was a great job. I fell in love with the residents and they with me. However, as always, everything must come to an end and so it did. The administrator thought she could save the company money if she cut my hours to part time just to do the scheduling and the residents could run the programs. This upset the residents deeply and they wrote many letters to the owner to try to get the decision reversed. But he wouldn't budge. I could not exist on half my salary so I accepted another position and resigned.

CHAPTER 5

AN ADMINISTRATOR FROM HELL

I mailed out my resume to different facilities and went for a couple of interviews. I was told it would be about three weeks before either facility would make its decision on hiring so I went to Indiana for a two weeks vacation. While I was in Indiana I received a phone call there from the assistant manager of one of the facilities. She told me the administrator was on vacation, but they had discussed my qualifications and she was instructed to offer me a position.

I went to my new position with hope that things would work out for the better. This was a facility in one of the most prestigious and wealthy areas in southern California. It was a beautiful facility where the clientele included wealthy retired writers, actors and artists. In the beginning it was great, for not only was I making a good salary with great benefits, I had a budget of eleven-hundred and forty dollars a month and a twenty-one passenger bus for outings.

I knew I had some adjusting to do considering the type of resident clientele there, but figured people are people. I would be able to run a program designed to their interests with very little change in the agenda and contacts with whom I had worked.

I attended their town hall meeting and requested volunteers to be on scheduling committees for both the in house activities and programs away from the facility. In the committee meetings I would present them with ideas about programs and outings. Then the committees would present suggestions and after discussion the committee voted on what should be scheduled.

Besides the places they were accustomed to going such as the opera, theatre, ballet and cruises I added horse races, educational facilities, sight seeing, museums, several out of town unique restaurants for lunch and shopping trips.

While we were on route we played games and sang. Different ones also shared stories about their past experiences.

One of the residents was a ninety year old lady who was as, the saying goes, quite a corker. She had family friends that were on the Titanic and she shared memories with us on one of the outings. When we reached our destination she was the first one off the bus and walked so fast it was hard for the rest to keep up with her. On one occasion I asked her if she had any children and she responded, "No not yet!"

With each outing I received positive comments and they would add "You have provided us with programs and outings to places we have never been and it feels so good to have fun and let our hair down once in awhile. Everyone else thinks all we want to do is act like a stuffed shirt."

Shortly after I began my employment the administrator returned from his vacation and I could tell immediately that he didn't like me. Although the residents accepted me and the activities were going great, the administrator felt I didn't have the social background to work with his clientele. He was the most difficult person for whom I have ever worked. He disapproved of me and everything I did and showed it daily.

For instance, I had scheduled a roaring twenties, Halloween costume party and had hired a group called the Parasol Strutters. Their costumes were from the era, they carried parasols and would get audience participation with their show. I told the administrator who I had hired and he stated he didn't feel that type of entertainment was suited for his facility, but it was too late to cancel so the program went as scheduled.

I had my husband attend to video the occasion as I felt the administrator might like to see how the program was accepted. The residents really enjoyed the entertainment and some of the ladies kicked off their shoes and had a ball.

The next morning I went into the administrator's office. He asked me how the party went and I told him what a good time the residents had. He commented, "You mean our residents enjoyed those flappers?" I told him they had a ball and I offered him a copy of the video of the party if he'd like to see it, but he said he didn't have time to watch it.

When outings or special programs were scheduled I would prepare a flyer, announcing all of the information regarding the occasion and cost if any. If reservations were required I included a sign up sheet. Every time I put up a flyer I would find it in my mail box the following morning defaced and notes written on it. One in particular was a free tour of Miramar Military base. When I arrived to work the next morning I found it in my box with notes asking, "Is Miramar one word or two and is this free?" I pointed out that Miramar was one word and yes it was FREE as written on the flyer in capitol letters. He then asked, "Well is it free for everyone or just you and the driver?" I exclaimed, of course it is free for everyone. If it wasn't I would not have listed it as such. These were just a couple of instances that occurred almost daily.

While I was in his office I said, "I really don't know what to do to please you. When I was hired I was told that I was here to satisfy the residents and the residents have told me they are thoroughly enjoying everything I am scheduling and have told me they have mentioned this to you each time they see you". With that he stated, "I really don't care what the residents want. It's what I want that counts." Bear in mind, the residents he didn't care to please were paying thousands of dollars rent monthly to live there.

I never knew what to expect when I arrived at work and I would get nauseous before I made it to my office. He made working conditions so horrible for everyone, several of the long time employees quit giving up their retirement benefits.

After eight months dealing with the working conditions it was becoming unbearable. So when I received a call with another job offer to work in a nursing home, I accepted the position with the stipulation that I would have to attend school for my certification prior to my starting date. The administrator agreed so I enrolled in school and submitted my resignation.

CHAPTER 6

NURSING HOMES, THE GOOD AND BAD

I attended the certification course and although I felt the classes were rather boring and I felt the activities they recommended were geared towards low functioning individuals only, I learned everything they offered, only to discover was next to useless. I received my certification and reported to my new job the following Monday.

I was so excited to be working with nursing home residents again that I could hardly wait for my first day on the job. I didn't know it then, but I was about to venture into a position that would be the most stressful position anyone could imagine. A position that required extra hours on the job and most of my time at home. When I was home I was either working on a fund raiser, craft project, a special event, completing paper work, preparing flyers or the activity calendar.

Had I known what I was getting into I may have sought employment elsewhere. By the time I realized my position was more than I had bargained for I had gotten to know several of the residents. I felt a real burden for them with the same compassion I had in my volunteer work.

I was fortunate with my first position because I had two experienced assistants, Verla and Toni who helped me get through my first few weeks until I knew where everything was and some of the duties of the position.

After meeting the residents and learning my way around I thought this won't be so bad, I can do this. Of course I hadn't gotten involved to any degree with charting of the residents progress or many of the other additional duties that were expected. When I found out what all was involved in running my department I was shocked. Besides running activities and attending meetings there was a mountain of charting. However, it wasn't as bad then as it is now.

I will never forget when I was told you have resident council today. Resident council! What was that? I didn't remember anything being mentioned about that in school. However one of my assistants explained that it is a meeting run by the more alert residents, with a president and in some cases a vice president to voice concerns or share positive comments regarding their care. The activity director had to attend to take minutes and assist in the meeting when needed. The only people allowed to attend are the residents, the activity director and the California State ombudsman "who is a patient advocate of the State." All others can only attend by invitation of the officers.

The activity director has to take all of the written concerns and problems to the various department heads of where the concerns are directed for a written response on how they plan to remedy the problems. My first minutes were as big as a book. I was told in the Resident Council meeting that the problems had existed for a long time with no attempt to correct them.

However, it wasn't until I had worked there for awhile that I found out why there were so many concerns preventing the facility from passing State survey inspections. It didn't take a brain surgeon to see that things were not right.

The facility was run so poorly that all departments had many deficiencies from the past several surveys. And even though they had deficiencies, the owner seemed to prefer to pay the fines for not being in compliance than to correct the problems.

The dietary department were only given $1.50 a day per resident for meals. The food was not only horrible it was served in a manner that looked like it had already been eaten. The activity department was only allowed $100.00 a month to purchase supplies, game prizes and pay for entertainment. The nursing department only had a couple of good nurses. The rest were lazy and the cleanliness of the facility left a lot to be desired. In fact the facility as a whole was one where you wouldn't send your worst enemy.

The facility was getting ready for survey and my department was under staffed. So I was allowed to hire another assistant. I hired

Lidia, who was an ambitious young lady with a lot of spunk and energy. A quality much needed in that facility because the activity staff had to do a great deal of the nurses duties. The nurses would not get many of the residents up and some that were gotten up were not ready to attend the programs. My staff and I would help get them dressed and make them presentable to attend groups.

Outings and outside activities were much the same. I couldn't get any help getting the residents outside and when an outing was scheduled the residents were never ready on time. The activity staff would have to help get them dressed. We were not allowed to take a nurse nor nurse's aid with us on outings. When a resident had to go to the bathroom or need a diaper changed the activity staff had to do it. They also sent the residents medication with us for the activity staff to administer. This is not allowed inside the facility by State Regulations. I couldn't understand why it was expected on an outing.

The nurses would not help or give care to any resident that had not been assigned to them. If we asked for help we were either ignored or told he or she is not my patient.

I recall one occasion we had been on an outing with one of the ladies with Muscular Dystrophy (MS). The transportation was late in picking us back up so the outing was longer than planned. By the time we returned this lady was exhausted and told me she needed her diaper changed and needed to lie down to rest. I pushed her to the nurses station and explained the situation to the nurse sitting behind the desk and asked if they could please take care of her. Thinking the situation would be taken care of I went out to the van to retrieve another resident.

However, two more times I saw the resident still sitting where I had left her. I asked her if the nurses had taken care of her and she said no. So I again asked the nurse to please see that she got help and I was told, she's not my patient. That's when I lost my temper and shouted, "I don't care who's patient she is. You are a nurse so see that she is taken care of now!" She got up and started pushing the resident towards her room so I thought the matter was going to be taken care of and went to my office to complete some paper work before leaving for the day.

After an hour or so I was headed out the door for the night and walked past the dining room and saw this lady sitting in there crying. I approached her and asked what was the matter. She said she was so tired and uncomfortable she could hardly stand it. So I asked if the nurses had ever taken care of her and she said no.

I don't know when I have ever been so upset as I was then. So I told her I would see that she got some help and went to the administrator's office where she was sitting with the director of nurses. I told her what happened and asked if they would intervene. The nurse got up and headed to the station, but the administrator called the station to warn them she was coming so they could get busy taking care of the lady.

There were times when the residents had not been changed for such long periods of time they would be wet to their knees. We would take them to the nurses station and ask that they be changed and a few minutes later the nurse would push them back into the group covered with a lap blanket. When we would check, they hadn't been changed. The nurses just covered them up thinking we wouldn't notice.

One of the activities was nail care. Many times when we would start to do their nails we found hardened feces had accumulated under their finger nails. This meant they hadn't been washed since their last scheduled shower.

Food related activities regardless if they were in house programs or outings were more of the same. The food was never ready on time and I would have to go into the kitchen and help in the preparation.

The administrator would not see that I got the help I needed on outings. I had to rely on what ever volunteers I could get to help. The administrator didn't even want to provide them with lunch when we went out for a picnic. She expected them to push a wheel chair around for hours and pay for their own lunch on top of it. So my staff and I would buy them lunch out of our own pocket so I wouldn't lose my volunteers.

The only way I could get anything done for the residents was to lose my temper and scream loud enough so someone would pay attention to me and get the job done. As you can imagine, I wasn't very well liked by the nurses, but I didn't care. At least I was getting some care for the residents so I just kept fighting on the residents behalf because I knew if I didn't look out for their welfare no one would.

CHAPTER 7

PREPARING FOR STATE SURVEY

I was unaware of the impact of not passing a survey. But I decided I would make my department the best possible. So I watched the already scheduled activities and how the residents were reacting to what was being offered. I realized the alert residents were bored and were only attending because there was nothing else to do. There was very little offered that was suited for them. Most of the activities were geared for the lower functioning residents.

So the next question was how was I going to change it? First of all I had to become more familiar with the mandated requirements of California State Title 22 in regards to what was required for nursing home facilities.

In doing so I found that a lot of requirements could be interpreted in several different ways. It would just take some imagination and the guts to try something new. Most activity directors don't want to put forth the extra effort to make changes.

The required activities fall under the quality of life portion. The activity programs that must be provided are A: Activities that are planned and designed to meet the individual needs and interests. B: To make life more meaningful, C: To stimulate and support physical and mental capabilities to the fullest extent, D: To enable the resident to maintain the highest attainable social, physical and emotional functioning possible, but not necessarily to correct or remedy a disability. These guidelines are followed by a list of required activities.

Although there are mandated requirements for all departments I was only interested in what would affect the activity department. If I was going to make the activity department the best possible I would have to go above and beyond the requirements. I would make sure my residents were provided quality adult programs for the high functioning and programs geared down to the lower functioning as well. Since these types of programs would require money that my budget wouldn't cover I started fundraisers to allow the flexibility for additional activities.

I decided to try some of the activities I had done in the independent living facilities. Because of wheelchairs some of the activities would be next to impossible. So I went to work and figured how some of the programs could be adjusted to obtain full participation with the nursing home clientele.

In addition to bingo that was already being provided I scheduled several new table and group games. Book review, bible study, religious services for all faiths, exercise, movies & popcorn, weekly entertainment. Easy crafts were also provided for the lower functioning and advanced crafts for the high functioning were introduced. Residents made items either to give as gifts or keep for themselves.

I purchased dice cups, card holders, large crossword puzzles, wheel chair exercise games, travel videos and I recorded new musical tapes. I scheduled Easter egg hunts, costume and Holiday parties, and craft bazaars where we would sell things we made. I also scheduled separate activities for the MS residents. The MS residents were very special people. They all had severe handicaps, but mentally they were 100%. Spending time with them and providing activities they could participate in was a very rewarding experience and I grew to love them dearly and I included them in any way I could to make them feel useful and needed. They felt pride in being able to work. This would not only have a positive reaction for the residents it would also help my department.

One of my fondest memories of working with the MS residents is of a young man who before he was stricken with this horrible disease was a star football player for his high school. He was a handsome young man with a personality that would warm the heart of anyone who came in contact with him. He spent a lot of his time sitting in the front lobby greeting people as they entered. He knew all of the visitors by name and everyone loved him.

Although he was severely handicapped he had such a positive way of communicating and making friends with the other male residents. I assigned him to encourage attendance of the men who

27

were reluctant to attend groups to come. He was good at it and brought several to the groups.

His disease caused him to be paralyzed from the waist down. The use of his hands and arms were failing, and it was increasingly getting more difficult for him to speak. It was becoming very challenging for him to participate in activities without a lot of assistance, but he never complained and was very appreciative of any and all assistance.

On his forty-first birthday I saw him sitting in the hall and stopped to talk to him and wish him a happy birthday. I didn't know at the time how old he was, so I asked him. In his weak voice and slow speech he responded, "guess"? So I said twenty-nine. He smiled and said, "guess again". I kept guessing until I finally guessed his age. With that I said, "you sure don't look your age, how do you stay looking so young?" He answered "Because I'm happy." I thought to myself, how could anyone be happy in his condition? After all he had been in a wheel chair most of his life, he was robbed of a life that others take for granted; his youth, the ability to walk, marry, have a family and he was at the mercy of others for his total care.

His answer, his courage and attitude made such an impression on me I think of him every time I get discouraged and realize how lucky I am.

At the time I was working with the United Way for placement of individuals who had to do community service as part of their sentence set by the courts. Their crimes ranged from ditching school to drunk driving. The ones that I most enjoyed working with were the high school boys because I would assign them to spend the days with my MS resident. They pushed him outside for walks they read to him and played trivia. I knew my resident would have a positive impact on their lives.

At the end of each day the boys would come in to sign out and would tell me how much they enjoyed their day. At the end of their assigned service each one told me how lucky they were not to be crippled like my resident and they all left the facility with a different outlook on their lives. They vowed to straighten up their lives and make the most of it in the future.

Another young male resident, also crippled with MS worked daily with the activity department selling raffle tickets to raise funds to cover the additional costs of activity programs that the budget didn't cover. This made him feel needed and gave him something to do and he considered it his job. I will never forget his comment when he found out the owner didn't like fund raisers and removed the table where he sat daily selling tickets. His comment was, "Well if she thinks she's going to do away with my job, she's got another think coming." He simply continued selling his tickets.

It's people like these two young men that keep the activity staff going. They have been dealt a raw deal, yet have such a positive outlook on life.

CHAPTER 8

MY FIRST STATE SURVEY

I had no idea of what to expect with my first California State survey. But I was about to find out. The survey was conducted by surveyors that had been in the facility many times because of complaints and a history of bad surveys. They came in expecting the worst and in most cases they weren't disappointed.

Going through survey was very stressful. The surveyors were rude, with a negative attitude and were totally unrealistic as far as the activity department was concerned. Some of their rude comments to my assistant, Lidia were overheard by the Social Service Director who volunteered to support me if I wanted to file a complaint.

After about two weeks they called in the department heads for a final drilling before their exit. I had been forewarned by the administrator not to try to defend anything they said about my department, but to just take any negative comments and say the matter will be resolved.

They started telling me their findings which included accusing me of not making an announcement for the afternoon activities. They then stated the afternoon program of a military band was unsuited for one of the residents because she was sitting in the activity with her eyes closed.

They questioned why I scheduled certain activities. They went through our attendance books and questioned how we could say some of our residents fully participated in activity groups when those residents had handicaps.

My temper would not allow me to sit quiet and take their remarks any longer when I knew they were wrong. So, regardless of the forewarning I had received by the administrator, I could not allow them to accuse me of untruths. I said, "With all due respect, perhaps you didn't hear the announcements because you were out of the building for a two hour lunch break when the announcements were made. Since the activity started at two o'clock, I personally made the announcements at one o'clock and again at one-thirty and my entire department went to the rooms and personally invited the residents to the program and we assisted them into the group. Secondly, the lady that you saw sitting in the activity with her eyes closed, is blind and always keeps her eyes closed." Then I stated, "As far as my reason to schedule certain activities, I schedule activities based on the residents assessment of their past and present activity interest of things they enjoyed in the past and what they still enjoy. I ask the resident council for input each month as well as visit individuals and question them on what type of activities they would like to see in the facility

31

and as far as our attendance records go in regards to the handicapped individuals fully participating in the activities, I'm sure you are aware, that if an individual is participating to the fullest extent of their capabilities, even if they need assistance, they are fully participating."

With my last response to their accusations and comments, they said, "That is all we need from you, thank you for coming."

The following day it was time for their exit meeting with the administrator and department heads to tell us their findings. The activity department had no deficiencies and the surveyors complimented the department for doing an outstanding job. I was pleased, but shocked to say the least, after what they had put me through the previous day and the fact that I spoke up in defense of my department.

The following day, I received a phone call from the supervisor of surveyors commending me for running an outstanding activities program. I felt very good about the compliments I had received as I had been told if the surveyors don't give a deficiency your department passed, but they never give compliments.

Following the survey I did write a letter to the State and reported the verbal abuse my staff and myself were subjected to and the surveyors were reprimanded.

The rest of the facility didn't do well as there were so many deficiencies the facility was placed on fast track. This prevented the admission of any new residents except private pay. The facility department heads were given a designated time to correct all of the problems.

With my department doing so well I was the recipient of many slurs from the nursing staff such as, "Activities think they are smart asses. They didn't get into trouble and they think they can't do anything wrong." Each time I received these comments I would respond, "No we don't think we're any smarter than anyone else, we just do our job."

A short time after that my department began to find documents missing from the charts. I'm sure after the smart remarks I had received, someone thought they could get us into trouble if we were found to not have all of our documentation in the charts. When I reported it no one would believe me and would say, why would anyone remove documents from the charts? They suggested perhaps the charts were dropped and they fell out or maybe they were placed somewhere else in the charts. So nothing was ever done about it.

It got so bad that we had to Xerox all of our documentation and keep a copy in the office. Every time we would find a document missing I would make a copy of the form I had in the office, write on it, "This is a copy, the original has been removed and it is missing." Eventually it stopped.

Unless you have been through a survey you can't imagine the amount of stress that is put upon you. Not only by the surveyors, but by other departments who know nothing about the mandated requirements for the activity department. Many feel that the State must be impressed with some type of activity going on all the time while surveyors are in house so they make demands. What they don't know or choose to ignore is activities must be scheduled with break times to allow the residents time to lie down to rest. Residents must also have their diapers changed, or be taken to the bathroom and get their hands washed before meal times. This also allows the activity department time to chart, do room visits and prepare for the next activity.

However, I have never witnessed residents getting their hands washed before meal times. Is it such a big job to put them down for a rest and get them back up again? Most do not do it and if they do put the residents down for a rest they are usually down for the remainder of the day.

CHAPTER 9

WHEN A FACILITY DOES NOT PASS SURVEY

When a facility does not pass survey and if the findings are severe, the administrator and department heads that failed are usually let go. If the findings are considered to be life threatening the facility will be given a citation. This incurs not only a huge fine, but the facility could lose its license to accept Medicare/Medi-Cal patients and could possibly close its doors.

This was the case in my first survey. The facility had failed in all departments except mine. They had to pay a tremendous fine and the administrator and several department heads were let go.

That is when I first met, Nel, who had been hired to replace the existing administrator. I was going down the hall to assist some alert residents to a called resident meeting and as I passed her, she reached out her hand, stopped me and asked, "Who are you?" I thought to myself, I just went through a horrible time with survey, now what's going to happen? We hadn't been told anything and had no idea the administrator was being replaced, but when we got into the meeting Nel was introduced as the new administrator.

The following day she came into my office to get acquainted and check on my department. She asked if I needed more supplies or assistants, who provided transportation and how many nurses or nurses aids were sent with me on outings? When I told her we never had a nurse or aid go with us she said, "Well they will now." And from that time on we never left for an outing without at least two nurses or nurses aids going with us. She had me put up a sign-up sheet by the time clock for any nurse or aid that was scheduled off on the day of our outing. They could earn overtime pay by accompanying us.

Nel took her job seriously. She was captain of her ship and let everyone know that if they wanted their job they would abide by the rules to present them selves in a professional manner both in their work and appearance. She didn't allow tongue rings or tattoos and if they had them they had better not be visible while on the job, especially if they were part of the staff that would be out on the floor. She demanded team work and got it. She was strict but fair to everyone and would go to any lengths necessary to make the work place better for her staff. If she knew you were doing your job she fully supported you and your efforts. Even though she couldn't get pay raises due to the facility's situation, she found other ways to show her appreciation for a job well done. For that she was loved and respected by everyone that worked for her. I found her to be the best administrator I have ever worked with. Although she had a very big job to do, she was never too busy to spend a few minutes with her staff to say hello or have a laugh. Every morning she toured the facility to make sure everything was okay and questioned the staff if they were having any problems that needed her attention. When it came to activities I received her total support both on indoor and outdoor activities. When we had a fund raiser going she was the first to purchase whatever we were selling. If it came to needing help to push a wheelchair outside for an event, she was first in line behind a wheelchair. Many times I saw her pushing a resident into an activity. Because she did it she demanded that all floor staff assist us in transporting residents to activities as part of their job.

Nel was not made aware of how bad things were at the facility when she accepted the position and didn't know until it was too late to back out of her commitment. She gave it her all trying to turn things around and hoped it would be enough before the return survey in three months.

There had been a vast improvement, but not enough to stop the wheels that were already in motion due to so many failed surveys in the past.

There is only one word to describe what happened next, and that is devastation. This was without a doubt the worst experience of my entire life in the work place. The facility was given a short period of time to transfer all of the Medicare/Medi-Cal residents to any other facilities that had openings. Every day, residents were sent out to other facilities by every ambulance company available and were being taken away several at a time.

The residents loved the activities, had made many friends that had become their extended families and didn't want to leave those they loved and what they called home. Everyone was crying and hugging their friends as they were whisked away. Everyday all day long they would cling to me crying and beg me not to let them be taken away. But there was nothing I could do but try to assure them that things would be okay. I promised each one that I would schedule my remaining outings to bring their friends for visits no matter where they were taken.

I would tell them goodbye as each one was loaded in the wheelchair vans, go into my office, cry like a baby, take a deep breath and go out to tell the next load goodbye. This went on for days on end until by the time the last remaining Medicare/Medi-Cal residents were gone I was totally mentally and physically drained.

In the meantime I had been getting calls from the owner to go to the sister facility which was also having trouble passing a survey. Their activity department had received several deficiencies in their last survey. I really didn't want to go as I had heard the facility wasn't run any better than the one where I was when I first arrived. So I kept stalling in giving an answer. Finally one day I was told that if I didn't take the transfer offered, there would not be a position for me. We agreed on my salary and I accepted the offer.

CHAPTER 10

THE SISTER FACILITY

I reported to work the following Monday and my fears were justified. It was more of the same as I had experienced before Nel had been hired in the previous facility.

I started off my position under adverse conditions as the administrator had been told by the owner that I had been hired, what my salary would be and she didn't have any say in the matter. She was not very trusting and she didn't show any support for activities.

My office was no larger than a good sized closet. Not only was this the place where supplies were kept, it was also where assistants, Geneva, Linda, Lee, Karen, Rhonda and I had to do our paper work. My staff had to use bedside tables for desk. Although there were other rooms sitting vacant that would have been better suited for my department, the owner and administrator would not allow us to use any of them.

Supplies were very limited and I had the same one-hundred dollars a month budget as I had in the other facility with twice the amount of residents. However, the administrator wouldn't give me the money up front. I had to ask for cash to go shopping for supplies and bring back the receipts with any change left to her.

They refused to pay for any entertainment. They felt I could get free entertainment. Entertainers used to donate their services until they found out they could get paid and started charging. The only people I could get were from schools and churches once in awhile.

They wouldn't allow fundraisers so I was very limited as to what I could accomplish. I donated some supplies, but the department had so little I couldn't afford to stock the department myself out of my own pocket. I had to make do with what we had and what little I could afford to donate.

After my staff punched in they also had to sign in when they reached the office. She wanted to know I wasn't allowing them to play around when they were on the clock.

There was a strict rule against over time so if employees didn't have time to complete their paper work at the end of their shift they were required to punch out and go back and complete their paper work off of the clock. This was a well known fact and although it is against the labor law it was expected.

Even though I didn't like working there, I decided I would do the best job possible under the restraints of the position until something better came along.

I revamped the department and scheduled new activities. Knowing the participation I had gotten from the advanced crafts class I scheduled and taught the class.

The first craft project was bean art. I prepared pictures of butterflies on cardboard and the residents were to glue the different colored beans on the picture depending on what color they wanted their butterfly.

One of the ladies who wanted to attend was blind. I couldn't imagine how she could do the project when she couldn't see the picture or color of the beans, but if she was willing to try, I decided I would find a way so she could participate. I asked her what colors she wanted in her butterfly. I laid the beans out in front of her in a position of clock hours and told her what color was at what time. I put the glue on the picture where the bean should be placed and put my finger next to the glue. She picked up the bean, found my finger and placed the bean along side of it. Much to my surprise, it turned out really good and she beamed with satisfaction over her accomplishments.

After the pictures were done I wrote each residents' name on the bottom of their art, took them outside and sprayed them with lacquer so they would not only shine, but they would not get bugs in them. Then I took each one their picture to see before I put them on display. When I got to her room I told her the pictures were done and I was getting ready to display them. She asked me to bring hers over so she could see it. I wasn't sure how she would accomplish this being blind, but I took it to her and watched her expressions as she ran her fingers over it as though she was seeing each detail. She smiled and said, "It's beautiful, thank you so much for allowing me to attend the class, I am thrilled that you are going to put it on display." That gave me such a since of pride that I was able to get full participation from a blind person in crafts.

I only worked there a couple of months when I received a call offering me another position. I made sure all of the charting was up to date, the calendar for the next month was completed and started putting up Christmas decorations on the day before I left so my staff wouldn't have to do it all by themselves. However, when I arrived for my last day there, all the decorations that I had put up were gone. I asked what happened to them and was told that the decorations weren't where the administrator wanted them put as they were not where they had always been. They were removed by the maintenance department. So my staff had to put them all up anyway with the administrator's supervision. So with that, I said, "fine I don't really care where they are put as I won't be here to see them anyway" and spent my last day visiting the residents.

I enjoyed my staff and really hated to leave them, but Geneva came to work for me in another facility and was still with me when I retired.

CHAPTER 11

OUT OF THE FRYING PAN INTO THE FIRE

This was another facility where the activity department could not pass survey and I had been recommended to the owner/administrator by his director of nurses with whom I had worked previously. She told him that I would not only meet the expectations of the position, but would exceed them and I would pass survey.

We had several phone conversations and I interviewed with him before I accepted his offer and he talked a good story of how he felt about the importance of a good activity department and how much he needed someone that could pass survey. He said he didn't have a set budget for the department, but if I needed anything all I had to do was let him know and he would see that I got it.

My office wasn't even a room. It was an exit that had been sealed off. I had a lot to do to get ready for survey so I piled things so I could get through to my desk and began my task of organizing the office procedures and policies. I also trained the staff, got all of the charting up to date, revamped the entire activity schedule and was ready for surveyors prior to their arrival date.

I passed the survey with flying colors, but the rest of the facility didn't do so well. They were given three months to correct the problems before the surveyors returned. They finally did pass survey with just a few deficiencies and all that was required was a written plan of correction.

After the return survey was over, the owner felt he had another year before the survey was due again so he wouldn't get the supplies I needed. He wanted me to give fruit out of the kitchen for game prizes. I spoke with him and explained I felt I could get better participation if I could give a small prize in place of the fruit. I told him that I could purchase small items that would be very inexpensive. He said I could do that, but he wanted me to pay for the things out of my pocket and bring him the receipts. He would reimburse me the following pay schedule. I didn't like the idea, but went along with it for the residents' sake until I could get some fundraisers going to cover the supply cost.

Getting the money to pay the entertainers was another challenge. I would have to submit a request for payment before the end of the month for the following month's entertainment schedule. I did that with several follow-up requests yet he still hadn't given me the money when the entertainers arrived. So I would have to go to his office again to request payment and was usually told he could not be disturbed. Some times the entertainers would end up barging into his office and demanding payment.

Most of what went on in that facility was no better than my first facility and in a lot of areas it was worse.

The food was horrible, the place was alive with roaches and most of the staff were on drugs and were stealing the residents medication if it was something that would make them high. The residents were not getting quality care at all and when they reported it they were ignored.

Needless to say, our pre-employment conversations were only to get me to accept the position because he needed his activity department cleaned up. After the survey was over he could relax and show his true colors. I could see it wasn't going to get any better, so when another job offer came in I resigned.

CHAPTER 12

MOVING ON UP

Moving on up was right as my office was on the fourth floor. It wasn't much larger than where I left, but we had our own bathroom, a couple of closets and a small storage place for supplies. The facility was clean and the employees were friendly and I had a decent budget to work with. That was a plus in itself.

When I arrived at my office I was treated like a queen. My staff, Joy, Nikki and Phyllis had the office decorated with balloons and welcome signs. They were hard working, dedicated and totally qualified. All they needed was some direction. The administrator was Nel, who was the best administrator anyone could have. So I knew I would be happy there.

After a few months I brought my previous assistants, Geneva and Verla aboard and hired Marvin. We made a great team and we enjoyed working together.

The residents were lovely and very excited to begin the new activities that I mentioned I wanted to try. And of course as always with my previous experiences, I again scheduled advanced crafts and' like before, I had good attendance and participation. We did many projects, from seasonal decorations to wearable art. One we did that turned out to be a master piece was a facility quilt. Each resident was given a section to sew together. Then my friend Jeanie, secured all of the sections together by machine, and monogrammed each person's name on the section they had put together along with the facilities name and the year it was completed. It turned out beautifully and hung on display long after I left the facility.

Some of my favorite memories and most rewarding experiences there were working with the handicapped and a lady with Alzheimer's. The lady had such a short attention span we couldn't get her to stay in activities for more than a few minutes and she would wheel herself out. Except for the advanced crafts. She needed very little direction. Everything she made was exceptional and she would stay in the class until it was over one to two hours later. When we made necklaces she made three or four and would wear all of them at the same time.

Another lady who was younger than most of the other residents, had suffered a stroke and was going through rehabilitation to try to regain the use of her arm and hand. She wouldn't come into activities because she thought she was much younger than the others and she didn't think she would enjoy it. I began visiting her almost daily and invited her to the craft class. I felt if she would attend one time she would enjoy it enough to come back. I explained that I had other residents attending that were about her age. Besides working on crafts we enjoyed adult conversation and socializing. Closer friendships resulted from our mutual sharing.

She commented that she had never been artistic and doubted if she could do any of the projects as she only had use of one arm and hand. So I told her the stories of my blind lady and of a lady who attended with limited use of both arms and hands due to M.S. I also told her I would help her and if there was anything she couldn't complete, I would complete it for her.

It took two weeks before I could convince her to attend. As I expected, she enjoyed the class and was able to do a lot more than she thought she could. She started attending all of the programs. After she had been coming to the craft class a month or so, she felt she was getting more therapy in my class than in the therapy sessions. She invited the therapist in to see what she was doing. He did come in and watched her and agreed she was getting the therapy she needed in my class. It wasn't long before she had gained most of the use of her hand and arm.

My class had grown to the point where I had to have one or more of my assistants come in and help me. Besides ladies I had some men attending so I also began a men's work shop.

One of our residents was a young man who was paralyzed from the waist down and had suffered severe burns on his legs and buttocks because his private care giver had sat him in a tub of very hot water. I persuaded him to attend both classes if for no other reason than to fill some lonely hours. He really enjoyed both of the classes and then started attending other groups.

Months after he was discharged he came back to see me and to thank me for persuading him to come to my classes. He said that because of my persistence he found out he could do a lot more than he thought he could. For that alone he would be eternally grateful.

During the Holiday season each wing made decorations for the Christmas tree in their station's dining room. On the station for the more disoriented my assistant Marvin, who was assigned to that station was helping the residents string popcorn. The residents were seated down each side of a long table. The more alert ones in the group would put a needle through the piece of corn and than push the kernel down to the next one and that person would push it to the next one and so on. After some time had passed, my assistant, Marvin realized that one side of the table didn't have much popcorn on their thread. He started watching them more closely and found that when the popcorn reached the last lady, she was pulling it off of the thread and eating it. So with that he decided he needed to sit the lady who was eating their decoration away from the table and find something else for her to do.

Another amusing story in that facility was when I had to have the piano tuned. There was no other place to have activities other than where the piano was, so I had to schedule the piano tuning at a time when the noise level of the activity would be lower. I scheduled it during the same time a table game was to be played.

Prior to the time of the scheduled tuning I informed the residents that the repairman would be tuning the piano during the activity and asked them if it would interfere with their game. They all agreed it wouldn't. However, one lady either didn't hear me or get the concept of what I had told them. About half way through the tuning with the repairman striking each key several times while tightening the strings, one of the ladies leaned over to the one sitting next to her and in a loud enough voice that everyone in the room over heard she exclaimed, "I've been listening to that man for over half an hour and haven't recognized a song he's played yet!"

Then when the repairman was ready to leave I went up to pay him and the same lady, again very loudly said, "I don't know why she's paying him. We've had a lot better piano players than that."

The repairman laughed and as he left he told me that she had made his day and he couldn't wait to get back to the shop to tell her comments. I could hardly keep my mind on my driving going home that night because I couldn't get her comments off my mind. I laughed hysterically about it all of the way home. Even though years have passed since that incident I still have to chuckle about it every time it comes to mind.

Parking at the facility was a challenge as parking for staff was very limited. If you didn't arrive at the right time you'd have to park on the street and plug the meter. On one occasion I had to park on the street with a trunk full of supplies. So I asked my staff to keep their eyes open for a spot to clear so I could go out, move my car and unload the supplies.

My assistants, Verla and Geneva were in the process of taking some residents out for a stroll when they spotted two parking spaces open up. Geneva pushed her wheel chair in the space nearest the door while Verla came to tell me about it. Before I could get my car back to the lot, a young man pulled in the lot and tried to park in the spot near the door. Geneva would not move the wheelchair and pointed out the other space and the man reluctantly moved his car around to the next row. However, unbeknown to her, he was a big shot from the corporate office.

The activities were going exceptionally well. The residents were happy and we had passed survey with flying colors. Then the owner hired a new management company which felt they could save some money by discharging the administrator and replacing her with someone with less experience.

From that time on it was hell to work there. The corporate person who was sent down to discharge the administrator took over the administrative duties while interviewing for the position. He was rude and was bent on making everyone's life miserable. You've seen this type I'm sure, "I am the boss and don't you forget it."

And wouldn't you know, he was the same man that wasn't allowed to park in that space nearest the door.

Later that afternoon he called the department heads in for a meeting and told us Nel had been dismissed. While scanning the audience, he mentioned the parking lot incident stating, "when he arrived earlier that day, someone had pushed a wheelchair in a parking space he wanted forcing him to park further away from the door. He then said, he didn't see the individual in the room, but he would recognize her if he saw her and when he did she would be reprimanded". Of course I told my assistant, Geneva to stay clear of anywhere he might be. I am happy to report my assistant was able to avoid having any further contact with him.

After interviewing a few prospective administrators he decided on a retired Navy officer with no previous health care administrative experience. Within a few days everyone knew he didn't know what he was doing. He tried to run the facility like the military and started his first day with a meeting stating pretty much the same things the corporate man had. He told us what he would and would not allow. In every department head meeting we felt like we had just been with a military drill sergeant. It didn't get any better.

He had all of the department heads in every meeting whether it concerned their department or not. We were in meetings from four to six hours a day and we were expected to do our eight hour day jobs as well. When he found out the nursing department hadn't been completing it's charting, such as dates and the name of the facility, all department heads had to go in on Sundays to complete the nurses charting. Next he started having the department heads work weekends as managers of the day.

All of the department heads were frustrated and complained to each other. However, they wouldn't go in together to complain to him for fear they would get fired.

I tried to get excused from some of the meetings that had no bearing on my department. He refused to excuse me from attending.

I was having to do most of my work at home on my own time and was becoming exhausted.

After about a week I approached him again and asked to be excused from some of the meetings and again he refused. Then a couple of days later he called me into his office and he had written me up for not being a team player and not wanting to cooperate with management. I refused to sign it as I felt I was not being allowed the time to do my work at the work place while being instructed to do everyone else's job. He said he couldn't understand why I was upset about having to attend meetings and said I was the only who had complained. I informed him I wasn't the only one who was upset about the meetings. I was just the only one who had the nerve to say something about it.

After that meetings were called with no advanced warning. He would get on the intercom and call for all department heads to report to the conference room in five minutes. It didn't matter what we were doing. We had to drop everything and attend a meeting that was only for his ego. He couldn't make a decision without input from us. Most of it was trivial and all of it was meaningless to our departments. He would manage to keep us in the meetings for up to an hour just to talk. Due to the lack of time all department heads had to devote to their duties, staff and residents suffered.

One time he called a meeting at the same time the resident council meeting was scheduled. I told him I would not be able to attend his meeting as I had to attend resident council. He instructed me to cancel the resident meeting. I asked him if he was sure that's what he wanted to do as resident council meetings were a mandatory requirement of the State. He admitted he did not know that and said I could be excused from that particular meeting, but not to schedule another council meeting without checking with him first. I explained that resident council meetings have to be scheduled the same day and time each month and have precedence over everything else and I gave him the schedule of the resident council meetings in that facility. The director of nurses backed me up and suggested he refer to Title 22 to confirm what we had said.

He evidently did research the requirements as he never asked me to cancel another resident meeting and in fact started attending them.

After about six months of working under those conditions, several resigned and I was a nervous wreck.

The least little thing would bring me to tears and I was unable to sleep at night. I went to my doctor and he put me on tranquilizers and stress leave. He also wrote a letter to my boss that I was headed for a nervous break-down and I would not be returning to work until he released me. The company sent me to their physiologist and he confirmed my doctors orders and diagnosis.

It wasn't long after I returned to work that I was offered another position, back in the same building where I first worked. I accepted the offer, gave my two weeks notice and resigned. The facility was under new ownership and new staff, but was still having problems passing survey and rebuilding occupancy. Having heard of Nel's background and history and her ability to improve occupancy and pass survey, the owner was willing to pay her salary request and hired her.

CHAPTER 13

GOING HOME

Nel hired people that she had worked with before. She knew with them on board the facility could pass a survey and build occupancy. I knew I had my work cut out for me as I was replacing an individual who had been transferred into the department from the social services department. He had no experience in scheduling and directing activities and the end result was the department failed survey. The charting was delinquent and the scheduled activities left a lot to be desired. However, I knew with the support I would have from Nel I could bring the department up to standards with some hard work and perseverance.

Reporting to work my first day was like going home. I knew my way around and some of the residents and I would be working with quality department heads and floor staff that I had enjoyed working with before. I brought my assistants, Marvin and Nikki with me and Geneva came aboard two weeks later. The atmosphere was relaxed and pleasant. Everyone knew their jobs and did it well.

We spent the next two weeks getting acquainted with the residents, reassessing their activity interest and going through charts and updating the paperwork.

The third week I focused on my staff and making changes in the activity schedule. I let one of my staff members go as she refused to follow my direction. The other two were good in their job, but needed their talents redirected where they would be most productive. Once that was done I introduced new activities.

One of the things I introduced was a shopping cart. One of our residents' son made me a three shelf wooded cart with wheels. I covered it with contact paper and stocked it with everything from eatable goodies to socks, hose and cosmetics. Then I made some tokens that the residents could use as cash to purchase items off the cart and they loved it. It gave them a chance to shop twice a week. After the word got out about the shopping cart, other facilities added it to their schedule of activities.

I scheduled new adult table games and group programs as well as activities for the lower functioning residents. And as always, I scheduled my advanced crafts class. We made almost everything out of recyclable items and I would either store their items for them so they could have Christmas gifts to give or to keep for themselves.

We made things for a craft bazaar and we raised enough money to fully pay for a dinner party with entertainment for the residents and family members. And gifts were provided for every resident.

We had carnivals complete with a fortune teller, games and a dunk tank. Residents Eva, Julia, Thelma, Faba, Ken and Annabelle assisted with operating the booths. The residents could try to dunk staff for free and the staff could try their luck for a fee. We made enough money off of the dunk tank to cover the entire cost of the carnival.

The attendance in all activities was rapidly growing. My craft class had become so large with both ladies and men attending I had to have two of my assistants help me with the class.

Once I had all of the new programs in place and special events scheduled we were ready for survey. The whole facility passed survey with compliments. I also received special recognition from the surveying team for having an outstanding department and schedule of activities.

It took awhile to rebuild occupancy due to the past history of the facility, but things were looking up and the occupancy was increasing.

My activities were going better than I had ever experienced in past facilities. We had enough alert high functioning residents that it made activities a lot of fun and I continued adding new programs. We had quite a few Spanish speaking residents who wanted to learn better English. Some English speaking residents also wanted to learn Spanish. So I started a Spanish learning class. After the class they played bingo where each number was called out in English and Spanish. It was quite a success.

One of our ladies was admitted to the facility for therapy while recovering from hip surgery. She enjoyed the activities so much, she decided she would like to make the facility her home. When it was time for her to be discharged, she sold her belongings and moved in.

That time of my career was very gratifying and I was very happy and comfortable in my position. I had a great administrator and staff to work with, each department worked together as a team. The feeling in the building was relaxed and everyone was happy.

Before time for the next survey the corporate office sent two men to the facility. One of the men we were told was the corporate administrator who was to be working with Nel to assist her. With the experience Nel had she didn't need an assistant. She knew it had been the practice of the owner to bring new administrators into her buildings before she discharged the current ones.

Everyone knew he would be our new administrator so Nel resigned. However, he was a very nice man with a professional demeanor and everyone liked him.

The other man was supposed to be the corporate marketing director. Some of us were told he made a huge salary, but I never saw anything he did to earn it. He did move some furniture and wall hangings and walk around in expensive clothing attempting to look important. He relied upon department heads to give him leads for marketing.

In the beginning I was uneasy with having a new administrator because I had lost an administrator I loved working with. With my past history of working with some very bad administrators, I wasn't sure of what to expect from him. It took awhile for me to feel comfortable and in turn for him to learn my capabilities and feel comfortable with me. However, we ended up having a very good working relationship. I found him to be one of the kindest men I have ever known who really cared about the residents.

I never did feel comfortable with or trust the corporate marketing director. I didn't feel he earned the outlandish $75.00 per hour salary he bragged about getting paid. At the same time staff who were paid minimal wages were getting hours cut. But someone had to pay his salary. However, his inability to produce must have caught up with him because one morning he was no longer present in the department head meeting. I'll say this for him, he sure knew how to sell the owner a bill of goods.

A few months after we had our new administrator it was time for resurvey. Although we had passed our last survey and things were well on their way in a positive direction, the new administrator brought in some excellent staff that he had worked with previously and when it was time for survey we were ready. We passed survey again with flying colors and the surveyors gave me a $50.00 cash donation for my department.

Things were going well. Activities were well attended, residency kept increasing and we were getting recognized as being among the top five facilities in southern California and the best in our area.

I continued to introduce new programs and one of my assistants thought it would be fun to put on a show for the residents for Valentine's day. My assistant Shannon and I made the costumes and the show turned out pretty good and everyone involved in it had a lot of fun. So when it was time to plan something for Halloween, we put another show together and everyone enjoyed it including the performers.

Then some of our residents wanted to be in a show and asked me to organize another one. We decided it would be a Roaring Twenties show. My volunteer, Patty, my assistant, Shannon and myself made the costumes, of flapper dresses, head dress, arm bands, ties and hats. Resident, Mary assisted in alterations and I purchased spats for the men.

I purchased old records for the music of the 20's era and copied the songs to cassette. Our exercise instructor Lois, my assistants Shannon, Taynaya and myself choreographed the dances.

The cast of thirty consisted of the entire activity department, Geneva, Marvin, Shannon, Tanaya, Anna, Nicole, Barry and myself. Others were social services Susan, business office manager Jose, marketing director Patti, receptionist Martha, nurses Yolanda and Jeannie, house keeper Debbie, maintenance supervisor Jeff, volunteers Patty, Kathy, Carmen, Sylvie, Vanessa age 12, Ronnie age 6 and Johanna age 4. Adult Ed. instructors Lois and Tom. Residents in the cast were Eva, Sally, Mollie, Joan and Ken.

After a lot of practice the show turned out extremely well and we ended up taking it on the road. The money we earned for the show was donated to resident activities.

All of the performers were excellent. One of the high lights of the show was a number performed by our eighty-five year old, under five foot resident, Eva and our two little girls Ronnie and Johanna.

In my last place of employment, I had one of the best staffed departments I have ever worked with. They were conscientious and we had a good mixture of personalities that helped us get through many rough times.

Marvin was the department's comedian and brought many smiles and much laughter to residents and staff as he danced and sang along with the musical entertainers. He pushed the shopping cart around the facility sporting a crazy hat, wild wig or silly glasses while singing a song he made up as he went along.

Shannon was our quiet one with outstanding performing and artistic abilities that proved to be most valuable to the department on many occasions.

Geneva was one you could set your clock by. Not only was she the most dependable employee I ever had, she was our peace maker, house keeper, staff party planner and went out of her way to help everyone.

Anna had the ability to reach residents regardless of their mental or physical status with exceptional charting ability and she was mentor for information for her co-workers when I was unavailable.

Tanaya transferred into our department from nursing. She learned the needed skills with exceptional speed. She had a pleasing personality, was an excellent performer and added pizzaz to our show and performed her duties with a smile.

Nicole was a no frills type of individual that believed if there was a job to do, get it done now and talk about it later. She cared very deeply for the residents on her station and always looked out for their welfare. When it came to resident parties she put her whole heart into making it a time to remember.

Merley was a quiet type, but stood out in her ability to provide comfort and encouragement to the bed bound residents.

Barry was our practical joker who always kept the staff and residents on their toes. He loved working with the residents and was able to achieve tremendous participation results. And he had the ability and talent to fill in for cancellations from entertainers and religious services.

Although each one had special talents and unique personalities they worked together as one, sharing responsibilities and fun. All were very competent and were a real team.

The business office manager, Jose and the marketing director, Patti, were exceptional in their support of resident activities. They not only donated cash and items for the department on many occasions, they also volunteered their services to be involved in fund raisers and special events even though they had their own busy schedules.

Administrator Henry and other department heads of nursing, dietary, maintenance, housekeeping, medical records, care plan meeting coordinator, and therapy were all very supportive and willing to lend a hand.

Only one department head was unsupportive and went to great lengths to be negative. She accused me of several untruths and spread rumors to anyone who would listen.

She found fault with everything my department did and tried to supervise my staff. She made a statement that activity directors were a dime a dozen. However, she didn't say "good activity directors" so I'm sure she doesn't know the difference. The truth is, good activity directors are few and far between. Because of the stress of the position. Most of them have left the field and gone into different areas such as marketing, nursing or social services. Some have even left human services totally and have gone into the private sector in business.

I had two very devoted adult education instructors, Dr. Tom Craven and Lois Schenker. They both went far above and beyond the call of duty to assist in resident activities. They even volunteered their free time to help by performing in the shows and assisting with special events. Dr. Craven also provided room visits for those who were unable to attend groups and played Santa at Christmas.

On one occasion when Tom was providing room visits he went into the room of a terminally ill resident that kept clinging onto life as though he just wasn't ready to go. Tom asked him if there was anything he could do for him. The resident responded, "Yes, you could get me a "Coke"." So with the nurse's permission he returned to the resident with the requested beverage and held the can while the resident gratefully and eagerly consumed it. A week later he arrived to visit the male resident, but was told the man had died less then an hour after he had left him. It seemed that the man was waiting to enjoy his last "Coke" before he left this earth.

Several residents were very involved in the activities and assisted the activity department in many ways. A young man named Faba sold raffle tickets and he, Liz, Eva, Annebelle, Julia, Thelma and Ken assisted in our carnivals and craft sales. And Elizabeth who was a retired minister, preached when our church canceled.

One of our residents, Sally, went out of her way to befriend a new resident who was a very sweet Spanish lady who spoke very little English. The Spanish lady was so happy to have a friend in her new home she took her new friend a gift of some kind almost daily.

Another resident with Alzheimer's enjoyed going out often for a cigarette. On one occasion my adult education instructor, Tom, asked him how he was able to cover the cost with the price of cigarettes being so expensive and he replied, "I know they are expensive, but my brother buys them for me. He's a hired killer and makes a lot of money." Tom was so startled by the comment he asked, "What do you mean your brother is a hired killer?" The man very seriously answered, "He's an exterminator."

During another of Tom's activities, the residents were asked the question, "How many loves have you had during your lives?" One of the ladies answered. "I have had 223 loves in my life, but the last one was the best one. It was Jesus Christ."

Joyce M. Poxon

During an activity for the Alzheimer's residents, my assistants, Barry and Darci, would tell a story stopping intermittently to ask the residents questions or to recite the next line. One in particular that comes to mind was a story about a man's car stalling and he needed a way to get it pulled to the garage. No other automobile was anywhere to be seen. The man looked in the nearby pasture to see if there was a horse that he could hook up to his car, but all he saw was a goat. So the goat was hooked up to the car to pull it to the garage. The question to the residents was, "How do you think the man was able to get the goat to pull the heavy car?" One little lady responded with, "He gave it an enema!"

We also had some embarrassing yet amusing times and incidents. On one occasion my assistant, Barry volunteered to tape movies for us from HBO for our movie matinee. He was taping Beethoven 2 for us to show the next day. He fell asleep during the taping and the next morning he rewound the video and brought it with him to work. When it was time for the movie, my assistant, Geneva, put in the movie and went to the nurses station to do some charting. After an hour or so she was approached by one of the nurses who asked her what type of movie she was showing the residents. She responded with "Beethoven 2, why?" The nurse said "Well that's not what's playing now!" So she went into the TV room to find several nurses and residents watching an adult X rated movie. Geneva immediately stopped the video. One of our residents who was engrossed in what was on the screen hollered, "Why did you turn that off?, I was enjoying that." What had happened was after Barry went to sleep an adult movie came on. Since he didn't have the time to view it before bringing it in he was totally unaware of all he had taped.

Another time we had an incident when a family of a deceased male resident insisted on taking Dad home for an Irish wake. The administrator explained that he could not release the body to anyone except the undertaker as other prior arrangements had not been made. Thinking he had made his point clear, he left the room so the family could have time with Dad to say their goodbyes. However, the family closed the door and managed to get Dad dressed and pushed him out the window, carried him to the car, sat him in the seat, buckled him in and drove off. No one was aware of what had transpired until a nurse arrived for her shift and questioned if the resident's health had improved she was told the resident had died. The nurse said, "Well I just saw his family pull out of the parking lot with him sitting in the car." They ran to his room and, sure enough, he was gone. I've heard of grave robbing, but never heard of a corpse being stolen before they got to the grave! However, eventually the body got to the mortuary and received a proper burial. It never ceases to amaze me the lengths people will go to achieve what they want.

CHAPTER 14

CHANGES, CHANGES AND MORE CHANGES

There is one thing for certain when you work in a nursing home; you will go through many changes if you work there for any length of time. If the owner thinks he or she can make more money they will revamp an entire facility regardless of who gets hurt in the process. This means everyone including the residents.

And so it goes. Someone told the owner that big money could be made by eliminating the assisted care unit and putting in a sub-acute unit in its' place. Residents that were able to take care of themselves with little assistance were asked to move to other facilities.

Some of them accepted the move with little resistance. To others it was more of the same devastation I had experienced in my first nursing home position.

Three of our more alert residents were moved to a near by facility that was not run well at all. The facility had three outbreaks of scabies in a short period of time. Very few activities for the alert and higher functioning residents were offered.

In an effort to ease the blow of the move, I would go and get the ladies on advanced craft night and bring them to the class. They could continue with their projects and visit with their former fellow residents and friends.

I tried to get them to get involved in the activities where they were, but they told me there was nothing for them to do and they hated it there. So I picked up an activity calendar on my way out and took it home for review to high light activities I thought they would enjoy.

When I looked at the scheduled activities that evening I couldn't believe my eyes. They were only being offered three different activities a week. The rest were the same programs with a different title. They didn't offer quality entertainment. What they had was offered only once a month. No wonder my ladies and man were so unhappy!

Each week when I picked the ladies up I could see them going down hill very quickly. They had lost weight and looked drawn and were so unhappy it broke my heart. The man refused to eat and one of the ladies passed away a few months after she was moved there.

I have seen this happen many times when people are not happy and given some enjoyment to keep their minds and bodies active they deteriorate quickly.

My heart ached for them. At the same time I was totally fed up with facilities and owners who really don't care how many lives they destroy in order to make a buck.

There should be a law to prevent this. Heaven knows there are rules and regulations for everything else.

If I had the power, I would stop this sort of thing from happening. But since I don't my only consolation is to believe that what goes around, comes around. Someday owners and administrators of facilities all over the country will get paid back for all of the wrong they have done to innocent elderly people and the employees who try to make life better for them.

In the last couple of years before my retirement, nursing shortages were felt in every facility and hospital. If someone called off or didn't show others had to work doubles. The director of nurses, the quality assurance nurse and other licensed nurses who were working in other departments had to work weekends and overtime to cover the shortages on the floor. At times the staff looked more weary and unhealthy than the patients.

The sub-acute unit opened and patients were brought in most of them were on life support machines and a couple were comatose. Work loads were doubled. The stress level on the staff increased and all departments suffered.

As far as activities were concerned, it required mostly room visits. For those in a comatose state it's like providing activities for the dead. But that doesn't matter to the State. We still had to provide some sort of stimulation such as reading aloud, talking to them or applying lotion.

When surveyors returned for our third survey we had around fifteen in the unit. Yet with a lot of hard work from everyone we passed survey again. The activity department not only passed, but with compliments and a larger cash donation than I had received the year before.

I was told by my consultant that she had only heard of one other activity director that had received compliments and a cash donation. So I would have to say with the recognition I had received over the years and the ability to pass every survey with compliments I must have been doing something right.

Throughout the years I have worked with some excellent co-workers who knew their jobs and worked hard to make things better for the residents. There were a few however who thought they knew more about my department than I and did not hesitate to let me know. Quite often some would find fault while others tried to dictate what I should and should not do and even tried to supervise my staff.

Some young degree holders think they know how everything should be run. Experience shows they are the worst type of employee any facility could have because all they have is a piece of paper with no people skills or basic knowledge about how a facility should be run. This is especially true when others interfere with the activity department. It would be like me trying to run the social service department with my certification as activity director.

However, it has been my experience that ignorance, unprofessional behavior, inappropriate work place attire and a know-it-all attitude can be excused as being immature. It's the sad result of inexperience with a little dose of authority that has gone to their head.

This occurred in my last place of employment prior to my retirement. With the exception of a couple of co-workers in other departments who belong in the above category, I worked with some of the best in the field.

And the facility as a whole was run both efficiently and professionally with hard working, devoted and qualified staff.

My decision to retire early was in part due to stress in the department coupled with unnecessary pressure from others. With the loss of a long time employee and additional demands that were put upon me and my department from others I decided it was time to get out of the field while I still had my sanity.

As mentioned in the preface only the good activity directors suffer burn out. This is definitely true. Activity directors who are dedicated to providing the best for their residents feel they are being punished for doing the job they were hired to do. Very few in the health care field perceive the activity department as little more than facility baby sitters for the residents.

All administrators must make it mandatory for all departments to work together as a team for the good of the residents. The requirement for their activity staff to attend useless meetings must be dropped. Then I believe positive changes will occur. Everyone can assist residents when State surveyors are in house. So why can't it be a mandatory requirement all of the time? I have seen it happen. And it didn't cause the facility to lose employees because it was part of their policy.

I have been told on several occasions by State Surveyors that they know staff are just putting on a show for their benefit when they see staff coming out of the woodwork to push residents to and from activities. They have also stated to me that they know when they are not in house that the activity staff receive little help if any in transporting wheelchairs. At times this reflects on their decision making during a survey.

Activity directors don't feel they should be placed on a pedestal, but they do expect respect for what they are trying to do and assistance in accomplishing their goals. All departments should be trained to know that the activity department is a mandated requirement and part of the internal healing process and not a necessary evil.

Some of the other departments have to spend time with the residents to take care of their financial, personal or health care needs. Their schedules are not listed on calendars all over the facility. Therefore they are not on a time schedule as to when and where they have to accomplish their tasks.

The monthly activity calendar, however is on public display by law and our tasks have to be performed as scheduled. The activity department does not have the flexibility of schedule others do. Our publicly listed programs are posted for all to see. This rigidity does not apply to all other nursing home departments.

There is also an ego situation between activity directors because they are afraid another director might be able to do the job better. So when they leave a position they take most of the records with them. This is especially true if they have been fired. They don't want to make it easy on their replacement and be out done.

When I arrived for my last position everything was gone even the rolodex. However, I had been in the business long enough to know to keep an extra set of contacts at home so I just used my back up copy. You must provide three months of previous calendars to State surveyors of which were not left, but by the time the surveyors came in I was able to provide them with the needed calendars so I was okay.

A good activity director is an individual who is dedicated enough to go that extra mile to see that things happen and the residents are happy. The inner quality to produce results, can not be taught. It's as much a matter of the heart as it is of the mind.

It is a position that carries one of the highest percentages of stress and or total emotional breakdown compared to any other position in a nursing home. Not quite the reward one would expect for doing a good job, is it?

I don't see working conditions improving a great deal for activity directors. Many people either don't want to work or take the responsibility for their work. Therefore, the activity department often becomes the dumping ground for all other departments.

Without a unionized activity directors association to force facilities to make things better for their activity department conditions will not improve. Occasionally the consultants will make suggestions to the administrators, but the suggestions are rarely taken seriously. If ever an association needed a union, it's activities.

With all of this said, I do miss my friends, my staff, the residents and what I was able to provide for them. What I don't miss is the stress, aggravation and heartache that went along with it.

LET THE GUILTY STAND UP AND BE COUNTED

CHAPTER 15
STATE SURVEYORS

Years ago nursing homes were all run poorly. When you went in they stunk of urine, the residents were not kept clean, residents were tied in their wheelchairs and beds and nothing was provided for them to erase lonely hours or keep them mentally or physically stimulated. In short, a nursing home was a place where you wouldn't want your worse enemy. Something had to be done, so the State and Federal Government stepped in and made all of the regulations that are in affect today.

However, it is my opinion that the pendulum has swung too far in the other direction. Now State surveyors have the power to make or break a facility. Many surveyors use their power as a weapon to prove the necessity of their existence. If the surveyors don't find a problem then the Federal Government steps in and you get another survey from them because they feel the State didn't do its job.

Surveys would be acceptable by everyone if the surveyors found a problem and would work with the facilities to improve the care of the residents. But that is not the way it's done.

The State are the judge and jury. It makes facilities pay for not doing things the way they want it done. Surveyors put such fear in all of the employees everyone concerned is on edge for days or weeks while the surveyors are on site. The staff is under so much strain and stress sometimes it's almost unbearable. All of the employees are trying to stay a step ahead of what they think the surveyors are looking to correct. The surveyors attitude is one of accusation rather than helping assistance.

I'm not saying that surveys are unnecessary because they are. The goal is to keep things from happening like what happened in the first facility where I worked. However, it has been my experience that one of the biggest problems in nursing homes starts with the State and Federal Government.

I have been in surveys where the problems they found were ridiculous. For instance, one time we had a fire drill while they were in house. When one of the extinguishers was put back in it's place, it wasn't hooked on the hook properly and it slid down in the case. It was still very visible and accessible, but because it wasn't on the hook we were given a deficiency. Another case occurred when the recycling dumpster was full. We were waiting for the pick-up and before it was removed, the surveyors gave us a deficiency because there were flattened cardboard boxes laying on the pavement along side of the dumpster.

They can force a facility to take a Medicare patient even if the facility has had the patient before and knows that the family members or resident are so demanding it is impossible to please them. Or their care requires additional staff to lift them due to obesity or their handicap. Although the facility knows admitting or readmitting them would be cause for a certain deficiency during survey they have no choice in the matter unless they can prove they can't provide the care the resident needs. This is almost impossible.

When the State issues a citation they are allowed to assess enormous fines depending on the severity of their findings. This would be acceptable if at least a portion of the fines went towards the welfare of the residents in the way of a reduction in their share of cost or to purchase equipment or supplies to benefit the residents, but it doesn't. According to a nursing home official, all citation fines are deposited into a special state account to finance wages for administrators/managers in state receivership until sale/corrections are made at a facility and state control is relinquished.

When surveyors come into a facility they request the activity director to provide them with a list of the alert residents. However, they talk to other residents not on the list as well. Some individuals with Alzheimer's can be pretty convincing that they have all of their faculties.

Confused, dementia and Alzheimer's patients will fabricate stories about many things such as; We had a resident who told surveyors that the nurses hid her false teeth and wouldn't let her have them. The truth was, the resident didn't like wearing her teeth and took them out daily and put them in her drawer. They will also report being hit and tell it as though it's the truth. These same residents can't even remember if they've eaten. But regardless of what the accusation is, surveyors will more than likely believe the resident.

The State also goes overboard with what they claim is abuse or going against the resident's rights. If a resident refuses a bath or shower the facility can't bathe them, even if they smell so bad others can't stand to be around them. It doesn't matter if they are so confused they aren't fully aware of their surroundings and don't realize they haven't been bathed. What I don't understand about that situation is what about the other residents who have to smell them. Don't they also have rights? The nurses' only recourse is to try to convince the resident to have a shower, contact the family members to intervene and do a lot of charting as to why the resident has not been bathed.

State surveyors are totally unrealistic in many areas especially where activities are concerned. If a resident refuses to go to activities, the State sees the activity program as insufficient to satisfy the activity interest of the resident. Even though the resident has never been a social person and has always preferred solitude or self directed activities.

When a resident refuses to attend groups, the activity department has to provide activity room visits and do a lot of charting to defend their findings. The same goes for those unable to attend groups. Sometimes they just don't feel like being bothered and would prefer to rest or read a book. However, we still have to provide room visits and do a lot of charting to justify our rationale.

I have known of facilities which have been given a deficiency because a resident fell asleep during a program.

Their reasoning was the activity department was not providing the proper program to meet the individual needs of that particular resident.

If you can name one eight to ninety-five year old individual who has not drifted off to sleep during the day then you deserve a medal. Heck! I've known Senior Citizens to fall asleep during a conversation. After all they are old, tired and are not in good health or they wouldn't be in a nursing home to begin with. Come on, Get Real!

But because of the fear of a deficiency, some activity staff, will nudge, pat or call out the resident's name to keep them awake when surveyors are in house. Is this ridiculous or what?

Due to the amount of residents that have to be gotten up, bathed, dressed and fed they are aroused at the crack of dawn and when old people get tired, they are going to take a nap. I'll tell you one thing; if it were me in the nursing home and someone expected me to stay awake when I wanted to nap, I would tell them what they could do with their expectations!

It is also a requirement by the State that the activity department provide outings away from the facility. However, it's not mandatory that the facility provide the wheelchair transportation that at least ninety-five percent of the nursing home population needs. So it is up to the activity director to accomplish this feat. It used to be that ambulance companies would provide free outing transportation if the facility used their companies for other transportation needs to doctor's appointments and trips to hospitals. However, some of the nurses refused to call the companies that would provide the free service so free transportation kept getting more difficult to find and by the time I retired, all companies were charging for outings. And they would only provide transportation for six including the staff needed to push wheelchairs.

In all my years in the field I have yet to run across a State surveyor who was a former activity director. I think I met a recreational therapist one time, but that's like comparing apples with oranges. I know because I have replaced three recreational therapist, because they couldn't pass a survey. So like the saying goes, you can't judge someone unless you've walked a mile in their shoes.

All nursing home staff have so much paper work to do they spend about fifty percent of their time charting and ten to twenty percent attending mandatory meetings and in-services. So this only leaves about thirty to forty percent of their time to spend with the residents. If you ask a surveyor why they require so much paper work they will tell you they only require about three or four forms, which is a lie because if a resident isn't responding to treatment they are "triggered" which means another form or two has to be filled out.

To make things worse, facilities are so afraid that they won't cover everything that surveyors might want, they add additional forms to make sure all T's are crossed and every I is dotted. So the paper work just keeps increasing. Paperwork for its own sake.

When I retired my department had to fill out seven forms plus make entries on all other department's charting for each resident and if there was a change of condition it all had to be rewritten.

Then there were quality assurance forms that had to be filled out. And if a resident was sent to the hospital and was gone for more than seventy-two hours from most facilities it all had to be redone. Or if there was no change of condition an explanation had to be written as to why the charting didn't have to be redone.

It's time that the State and Federal Government wake up and smell the coffee. If their concern is truly the quality care the residents are receiving then do away with some of the paper work so staff can spend more time with the residents. Most of the deficiencies that are given are due to someone not charting the way surveyors want it. When they come into a facility they go through the charts with a fine tooth comb and everyone's paper work had better be correct.

CHAPTER 16

DO OWNERS REALLY CARE?

First of all nursing homes are businesses and the owners are in it to make all the money they can. If you don't believe it, why do you think there arc so many nursing homes around the country? In order to make the amount of money they want, most of them will not pay decent salaries to get qualified help or provide adequate budgets for the facility to operate on to provide the kind of care the residents deserve and for which they pay a lot to receive.

When I retired facilities on the average were charging Around $3,000.00 per resident per month. However, if the residents needed more extensive care such as a sub-acute unit the care was more costly. And in most cases the facility cost does not cover the cost of laundry or hair dresser. Medicare pays a per diem for Part A (Acute Care) coverage in full for twenty (20) days and per diem less Co-insurance for the remaining eighty (80) days or termination of benefits. Medi-Cal or the resident is responsible for the Co-insurance. Medi-cal pays

100% for services less "Share Of Cost" which is total income less $35.00 per month for personal needs. This includes personal items, clothing and cosmetics. When was the last time you tried to live on $35.00 per month?

Some owners and administrators count on the dedication of their activity directors and their staff, because they know a good director and their staff will see that they have the supplies needed to provide quality activities for the residents. Often they hold fundraisers or they will buy the items needed out of their own pockets. The end result is the activity department looks good because they have enough supplies. Yet no one realizes it's because of fundraisers and donations.

Then when the owners don't feel they are making enough money, the first thing they do is start cutting hours and the first department to be cut is activities.

They hire expensive management companies and have more highly paid corporate big shots than some retail chains.

If they didn't have to pay such big salaries to a whole lot of know little and do nothing people, they could pay their nursing home employees higher wages. In turn they could demand more qualified individuals and they wouldn't have to cut hours.

In most facilities there is no concern with over time during a State survey. Owners will pay what ever it takes to make sure their staff are on duty during a survey. In most cases after the survey is over, hours are watched more closely and at times staff's hours are cut. This is especially true if the facility passed.

Activity directors and their staffs get into the field because of their love and concern for the nursing home residents. They continue to work in the field because of their desire to make things better for those less fortunate. However, very few nursing homes realize or care about this devotion and their importance to the facility.

CHAPTER 17

ADMINISTRATORS

Although there are a few good administrators whom I have had the pleasure of working with, there are also some really bad ones as well. A lot of them try to pinch pennies by cutting back on supplies and equipment to save the owners money.

Another way they can cut back on expenses is to hire department heads fresh out of school with no previous experience and no people skills. They may have a degree, but base all of their knowledge on what they were taught in school. Therefore, their accomplishments include upsetting residents and fellow staff members and making everyone else's life miserable. Too often they are not reprimanded or counseled about their inadequate behavior.

Some schedule so many meetings that often staff members do not have time to finish their work and end up completing it off the clock. These administrators are aware of this and, even though it's illegal, they close their eyes and pretend it doesn't exist because the owner does not want overtime.

I had an occasion when my staff were upset about a situation with another department and needed to talk to the administrator. I arranged a meeting, but he put us off for several days. Finally when he did come in he hadn't ask the receptionist to hold his calls or tell her not to disturb him until after his meeting with us. He no more than got into our office when he received a call. After he hung up from that call he received another call. He said he had a visitor and left and never returned.

My staff were never given the opportunity to speak with him. They felt he could care less about them and showed no interest in the fact that his employees had concerns. The final result was my staff lost their respect for him and the morale level slumped for days.

These are the same type of administrators who can't find time for residents' family members. When doing research on prospective nursing facilities, if you request a meeting with the administrator and they won't take the time to schedule an appointment with you and keep it, run, don't walk to another facility. This will tell you they have no interest in you or your family member.

I recall when a male supervisor was forcing his staff to have sex with him during work hours. He told them if they didn't do it he would fire them. His staff were afraid to report it for fear that would also give him cause to fire them. It had been reported to the administrator by others who had witnessed it, but nothing was ever done about it.

In a facility where I worked, theft was rampant. One of our very alert residents had everything from clothing to money stolen from her. She begged the facility to try to catch the thief and I even volunteered to loan them my video camera to hide in her room so we could catch the one stealing from her. The administrator refused to do it, stating that he was afraid the thief could sue the facility. I think he just didn't want to pursue it for fear of what he might find out. Sure, the thief might try to sue, but could they win if they were caught on camera? I think they would have about as much chance of winning in court as a snowball would have of not melting in hell. What do you think?

CHAPTER 18

HOW GOOD ARE THE NURSES?

A nursing career in this day and age is a hard job if they are dedicated to their profession in providing quality care for their resident/patients. They have to work double shifts and several days without time off covering for others who call off or just don't show.

There are many nurses that could care less and get into the nursing field because it guarantees them employment and benefits because of the nursing shortage. Therefore if the facility does not have a qualified director of nurses (D.O.N.) and charge nurses that require high standards in the care their staff provides, the residents get neglected.

During my years in the field I have worked with some very bad nurses who didn't care about the residents and only did what they had to do and wouldn't do that if they could get away with it. On many occasions I have witnessed nurses and nurses aids sitting in residents rooms with their feet propped up on a bed watching soap operas.

The residents were ignored and neglected unless they were alert enough to realize they had not been given care.

There have been instances where nurses aids would get into an unoccupied bed and sleep or meet their girlfriend or boyfriend in the room and have sex. Many times housekeepers would find prophylactics on the floors or in the trash. In some cases suspicions were raised about sex with senile or mentally ill patients. It was too hard to catch them so rarely was anything done about it.

Some of the nurses and aids in some facilities were on drugs and would steal medication from the residents. Drug screening is rare in nursing homes because they are afraid of law suits. It can be quite expensive and involve some nasty publicity.

Some nurses were abusive to the residents. When they were caught or suspected of abuse and got fired they would just go work for another facility which does not screen their employees. So the abuse just goes on in another facility. The abuse that goes on can range from not changing residents for hours when they have soiled their diapers, yelling at the residents, threatening not to give care if the residents turn on their call lights to often, or putting their call light button out of reach, to throwing them in their bed or plopping them in a wheelchair. In rare instances staff have even gone as far as to hit the residents.

However, I must say at the last facility where I worked prior to my retirement, their nursing staff and aids were some of the best I have ever worked with throughout my career. Their licensed nurses had a good medical background. They were devoted, hard working and caring individuals who's main interest was to see that their residents got the best of care. These are qualities you don't find in very many facilities.

Part of this is due to the facility's screening process prior to hire. They went through a well planned training process and they had good department heads such as the director of nurses, a quality assurance nurse and caring devoted charge nurses.

CHAPTER 19

PROBLEM AND ABUSIVE STAFFING

Staffing can be a big problem in all facilities. The difference is how the facility handles these problems when they arise.

Some employees are more concerned about when they will get a break or when they can duck out to have a cigarette than they are about the residents. Some spend more time visiting and complaining then they do working.

Theft is a big problem in every facility. Not only are residents belongings stolen, staff will steal from departments and co-workers. I have had everything stolen from equipment to holiday decorations taken off the walls and Christmas trees. Other departments have had linens, equipment, tools and supplies stolen. Kitchens have had food stolen by the car loads, facilities have had framed paintings, chairs, tables, lamps and anything else that could be carried out the doors stolen. Residents have had their medication stolen as well as everything they own such as, radios, televisions, razors, cosmetics, jewelry, clothing and even underwear. Yes, I said underwear! This really happened in several facilities where I worked.

On one occasion, a lady had her under panties stolen. A few days later a housekeeper was bending over mopping the floor when her blouse slipped up and her slacks slipped down enough that you could plainly read the resident's name written across the back top of her panties in black marker.

Very few facilities will install cameras to catch the crooks because of the expense or they just don't care. Therefore, the theft continues.

However, in one facility where one of my assistants worked, the administrator decided to take drastic measures to stop the constant thefts. He purchased some rub off ink that glows in the dark, put it on several items including cash and placed the items in several different locations in the facility including residents rooms. Before time for the shift change he checked the places where he had placed the items. Finding they were missing, he called the police then called a mandatory all staff meeting. When everyone was in the room he turned off the lights. Much to everyone's surprise a housekeeper glowed from head to toe from handling the items then rubbing her hands on her clothes. He turned the lights back on, fired the girl on the spot. The police placed her under arrest and she left in handcuffs. Before he dismissed the staff he warned everyone that he meant business and would be repeating the same procedure as he saw fit and promised them if anyone got caught he would press charges. That ended the thievery in his building.

I'm sorry to say that it didn't happen in a place where I worked because nothing would have given me more pleasure than to see someone finally get caught stealing.

As far as cooperation with other departments goes, I have had bad experiences with most other departments at one time or another, due to a lack of cooperation, neglect of the residents or interference in what my department was trying to achieve failed because others failed to work as team members. But the department that gave me the most problems throughout my career was social services. Other activity directors have confided in me with similar experiences.

In all of my years in the field I have only worked with five social service people who worked with other departments as a team. One was director, Esther and her assistant, Aurora who were very supportive. Esther paid for a wonderful monthly animal program, "Kruzin Kritters". She assisted residents into activities and even purchased balloon bouquets for every resident on Valentine's Day. Another was an assistant, Doug who was very supportive.

Also assistant, Susan who always worked with activities from giving donations to performing in a couple of our shows. And assistant, Toni who transferred from activities to social services. She knew the importance of resident activities and would help whenever she could.

Although, I'm sure there are other social services staff that are team players, I haven't had the pleasure of working with them. Many feel they know how to run the entire facility and give instructions to everyone if they can get away with it. They try to down grade everyone's efforts, yet they don't offer any assistance. If you ask for help, they respond by saying that is not the job of the social services department. In most cases, you can forget about team work if it's the director of the department because most of them feel they are the entire team.

They will walk right past a resident in a wheelchair needing help getting in to the activity and won't take the time to help unless they are asked to do so. But they'll take time to criticize the activity staff or the person providing the program. These people are the type you would like to buy for what they're worth and sell them for what they think they're worth. Yet this is allowed to continue in every facility where I have worked.

In one facility where I worked, we only had the dining rooms for all of the activities including religious worship. The dining rooms also had to be decorated for all Holidays.

On Halloween the social service director took down all of the decorations as she felt it was inappropriate to have decorations up while services were going on. The end result was I had to put everything back up which was extra work that I didn't need.

Occasionally activity professionals leave for positions in social services work. They aren't so difficult to work with because they fully understand the requirements of the activity department.

CHAPTER 20

UNREALISTIC AND ABUSIVE FAMILY MEMBERS

Although nursing homes have their problems, the owners and staffing are not always the main concerns as family members can also be the problem in a nursing home.

It is never easy to place a loved one in a nursing home. It is one of the toughest decisions family members will have to make. For what ever reason, when a loved one has to be placed in a nursing home there is always a lot of guilt that goes along with it. This is especially true if the loved one being placed is a parent. Even if the family feel, they have done the best they can do. Because of an illness or handicap they may not be physically or financially able to provide the care themselves or hire home health care. They have no choice but placement in a nursing home.

So along with guilt comes denial. We do not want to believe that our parents' physical and or mental status has deteriorated. Therefore, some family members tend to turn into irate, demanding and impossible individuals to deal with. They demand that the same type of individualized care be given in a nursing home as they would have liked to have given at home. That is simply not going to happen as there are many residents to take care of and everyone can not be first or have a nurse at their side around the clock. That type of care would require a personal private duty nurse. And when they feel their parent is not given the type of care they desire, the first thing they do is call the State.

When the State is called the facility receives a visit from surveyors which causes additional stress on the staff.

When surveyors come in because of a complaint they not only look at the chart of the resident in question they also look randomly at other charts. If they find something that was not charted correctly they will charge the facility with a deficiency which could contribute to a fine. At the very least, the facility has to write a plan of correction and the State will return to see that the problem is corrected. So this starts the ball rolling downward.

When facilities are forced to pay fines, they have to recoup their losses. So the only thing that is accomplished is a reduction of hours of some of the departments. This only creates more shortages of staff to take care of the residents.

The sad part of it is, most nursing problems could be resolved if the director of nursing is contacted. And if there is another concern, or the nursing problem has not been corrected than the administrator should be contacted. Chances are neither one of them are aware of the problem. Family members owe it to their loved one and the nursing home to make the administrator and the director of nurses aware of the concern.

I'm not saying that the State should never be called. Usually unhappy family members have not reported the problem to the proper people to get the problem resolved before taking extreme measures and calling the State.

There is one thing to remember. When our parents are home they are the only ones we are concerned with. Living in a nursing home there are many people needing care. A nursing home is not the same as living at home and as much as staff would like it to be it can never replace living at home. With such a large population everyone has to have set times for getting up, for showers, getting dressed and eating their meals.

As far as activities are concerned, I have had family members demand that their loved one be taken into all activities. Even those that are scheduled for high functioning residents such as table games or advanced crafts. Some had advanced dementia or Alzheimer's to the extent they didn't even know where they were at. The family thought because they used to enjoy those things they could still participate. This is another case of denial and all that is accomplished is the parent gets frustrated because they can not keep up with the others.

There was an incident that was a case of denial to the extreme. The mother had at one time been a prominent person in her community with attachments to celebrities and people in politics. The daughter could not deal with what had happened to her mother and was laden with guilt because she could not take care of her. She was totally unrealistic in her expectations. She wanted her mother taken to bingo and the mother didn't even realize what was going on around her. So the daughter would bring her in and sit her at a table and play the game for her.

Another residents' daughter wanted a nurse at her mother's side around the clock. And when this didn't happen, she would go to the nurses station every time she visited accusing the nurses of abuse and lack of care and she reported her accusations to the State. The State visited the facility on several occasions to investigate.

However, the last time she called the State they were present when the full body search was done. The accusations were unfounded so that time there was no penalty. But the accusations continued.

Within a few minutes after the daughter would arrive she would go to the nurses station screaming and yelling that her mother wasn't being taken care of. Several times she complained that her mother was wet from one end to the other. The nurses couldn't understand how this could be because they had recently checked the mother. But would go back in to check again and would find the resident soaked from top to bottom and change her.

Finally one day a nurses aid was walking by the room after the daughter arrived and saw the daughter pouring the water from the bedside table on her mother! She immediately went back to the nurses station and reported what she had seen. This matter was resolved as the daughter was escorted out of the building and was told she could not come back.

However, she did come back during the evening when the regular nurses were off duty and had neglected to tell the evening staff that the daughter was not allowed to visit her mother or come in the facility. This time she went to the nurses screaming that her mother had a bruise on her hand. The nurse checked, but couldn't find a bruise. Later a nurse stepped in the room to assist the room mate and witnessed the daughter slamming her mother's hand in the night stand drawer.

The nurse went directly to the phone and in using the code called for male staff to come to the station to hold the daughter while the police was called. I was still on duty so when I heard the code call I also went down to the station to see what it was all about. The police took the daughter out in hand cuffs and that ended the problem with the abusive daughter. However, the staff had been put through hell with accusations of abuse.

I had heard of cases where a family member would bring a loved one near death to get attention. Or make it look like they were needed. They made a hero of themselves for taking care of a family member and saving their lives. Until that time I had never experienced it where I worked.

CHAPTER 21

ABUSIVE RESIDENTS

When I went to work in my last facility before my retirement, there was a young male resident who had been admitted from the hospital. His diagnosis was paralyzed from the waist down due to a job related accident. He constantly called the State reporting abuse with all kinds of outlandish accusations.

He knew the system and used it to benefit himself and cause the facility problems. He accused my department of not delivering his mail claiming he had written himself a letter which he never received along with some insurance checks. Of course this was a lie.

He made demands for me to purchase some costly art supplies for him. I explained my budget would not cover the cost and then told him I would be happy to go pick up the supplies he wanted if he would pay for them. He didn't want to do that and called the State and reported that I was not meeting his needs for self directed, independent activities.

He burnt the thermostat in his room with a cigarette lighter throwing the air conditioner out of order on the entire wing. He then called the State to report that the facility was not providing him air conditioning.

He would go out to the nurses station at night when the nurses were busy passing out medication. He would get his chart and write notes on the documents to substantiate his claims of abuse. Then he would scribble through statements that he didn't agree with and then call the State the following morning to report what his chart would substantiate.

With each report he made to the State, surveyors came out and wrote up the facility. When they looked in the chart it looked like the facility was aware of his claims of abuse and wasn't doing anything about it.

The fact that he had been making entries in his own chart could not be proven because he would initial the documents with the appropriate initials of his care givers. Although the care givers denied having written his statements, they couldn't prove they didn't do it.

They suspected he was the one making the entries, but they didn't catch him in the act. Until one night a nurse coming back to the station after her break caught him with his chart. They locked his chart in the med room so he couldn't get to it. Yet the facility suffered a lot of wrath from the State before they had proof of what was happening.

One day a male nurse was entering the facility at the same time with a female nurse to begin their shift. The male resident was sitting outside. As they passed him the resident threatened the female nurse with a statement that she had better keep her mouth shut about what had happened if she knew what was good for her.

When they got inside the male nurse questioned her about what the resident had said. She told him that the resident had tried to rape her. She was frightened of him and was afraid she would lose her job if she reported it as she didn't think anyone would believe her because of him being paralyzed. So instead, she, like the other female nurses that were assigned to him, requested a transfer to another section. They would not explain why other than they were afraid of him because he was mean and had a bad temper.

The male nurse convinced her to report what had happened and stated he would testify as to what he had overheard. She reported that while she was giving care he stood up out of his wheelchair, picked her up, threw her on the bed and would have accomplished his attempt of rape had she not been able to get away. When she reported the attack, several other nurses came forward and reported he had tried the same thing with them.

The nurses reports proved he wasn't paralyzed at all. It was a just an insurance scam and he was good enough with his pretense to pull it off. He had fooled the doctors and hospital with his claim of being paralyzed.

The end result was, the police were called and he was taken out of the facility in handcuffs. The last I heard he was in prison.

CHAPTER 22

NURSING HOME DOCTORS

Like everything else, there were some good doctors in nursing homes. But during my years in the business, on many occasions I have witnessed doctors arriving at the facility. They went straight to the chart, wrote their report and never even peeked in on the resident. Others would go to the residents rooms and stand in the door. They would look in at the resident and that was all they did. Yet they charted as if they had given the resident an examination. In reality they had only read the nurses notes and charted accordingly. Talk about Medicare, Medi-Cal and insurance fraud!

Other doctors don't come into the facility at all for months, even though they are supposed to visit monthly. I have no way of knowing if they bill for the months that they don't even show up at the facility. If they bill for non patient visits when they are in the facility I wouldn't doubt it.

Company paid physicals were a joke. The doctors examination of the staff consisted of listening to your heart, have you bend over and touch your toes and that's your physical.

CHAPTER 23

PROVIDERS OF HANDS ON CARE

Other departments besides the nursing give hands on care. The activity department is one of them which provides hands on care on a daily basis in assisting residents from one location to another and helping them get dressed. They comb hair, put on make up, do their nails and put on sweaters and lap robes. During outings assist the residents from pushing them in a wheelchair, assisting the ambulatory in walking, to hand washing and toileting.

Yet, when Medi-cal reimbursed facilities with extra funds there were stipulations put on the money that it could only be given to nurses who provided hands on care!

This stipulation has caused a lot of hurt feelings in other departments. They have felt they deserved to be recognized for hands on care as well. This is just another case of uninformed, unknowledgeable people running the show for the American public and State assisted Medi-Cal).

So all in all there are a lot of problems involved in working in a nursing home that are not easily corrected. This is due to stipulations, regulations and demands that are put upon facilities and their staff by people who have little if any idea of what is involved with the total care of nursing home residents.

CHAPTER 24

SUMMING IT UP

With my mother being in a nursing home in Arkansas, my volunteer work in Indiana, my employment in California, by visiting other facilities and talking to activity directors from other States, I can tell you there isn't much difference in the way nursing homes are run and State regulations all over the country. Therefore, it doesn't matter what State you live in, you still need to research the facilities before placement.

If you find a facility that has a good activity department where the activity staff are dedicated to their work, you can bet your loved one will be getting better care. This is because of their devotion to their work and compassion for the handicapped and elderly. They know how beneficial not only activities are, but personal hygiene and living conditions as well. They are like watch dogs for the residents and will go to any lengths possible to see that the residents are receiving the care they deserve and for which you are paying.

CHAPTER 25

PLACEMENT IN A NURSING HOME

The best advise I can give family members is if at all possible, keep your loved one at home. If you are unable to care for them yourself, there are home health agencies that provide health care in the home. You can find a number in the phone book to contact a home health care service. If you would like to hire a private duty nurse or nurses aid, ask the nurses in nursing homes. They may know of someone who might be interested in providing private duty care. Several nurses and nurses aids have gone into private duty. Some prefer private duty as they only have one patient to care for instead of several. Some also provide private duty on a part time basis.

If this is not within your financial means and your decision is for placing a loved one in a nursing home then you must be realistic as to their capabilities. If you feel guilty about nursing home placement, ask yourself if you can provide the physical and or financial support to give your loved one the care they need for survival. If the answer is no than you must accept the fact that you have no other choice.

Realize that nursing home placement does not have to be a permanent situation. If at a later date you find that you are able to take care of your loved one you can have them discharged. We had a resident who spent a couple of weeks with us at least two or three times a year while the family members were on vacation.

There is another option you might consider to ease the blow of finalizing the permanent move to a nursing home. You can place your loved one in a nursing home for a short period of time from a few days to a few weeks. You can go on vacation or just have the time to make your decision.

If this could be helpful to you, talk to your doctor and the nursing home you have selected about this option.

This might just be what it takes for your family member to adjust, to learn the facility, get acquainted and attend some enjoyable activities. You might find that they enjoy it there because they have things to do and people their own age bracket to talk to that share some of their same interests.

Your loved one may have been placed in a nursing home and is able to get out of bed. Yet he or she chooses to stay in bed or sit alone in their room and you want them to be more actively involved in what the facility offers. Then try visiting more often and encourage them to attend activities and attend some activity groups with them.

Request that they be taken to the dining room for meals. Order a meal tray for yourself and eat with them a few times. This will not only give you an idea of what is being offered in programs but also the quality of the food. It will also help them learn their way around, meet other residents and accept their new surroundings.

Although the activity staff invite and encourage all residents to attend programs sometimes residents refuse and it takes a family member to get them involved. Tell the charge nurse at the station and the activity director that you want your family member to attend activities and remind your loved one each time you visit that you want them to attend.

There are activity programs designed for residents according to their mental and physical abilities. It's best not to force them to attend an activity that is beyond their mental capabilities as it will only frustrate them. Trying to compete with those who are more alert with higher functioning abilities can be very frustrating.

If you think your loved one has advanced dementia and would like more information on dementia and Alzheimer's disease, contact your local Alzheimer's foundation. They have literature available to help you understand more about these diseases.

CHAPTER 26

GUIDING YOU THROUGH YOUR RESEARCH

1   Read the most recent survey report that will be posted in the
        facility, usually close to the receptionist desk. If you can't
        locate it ask where it's posted. However, if you have never
        read a survey report the way they are written could be
        confusing and in some cases misleading. Bear in mind survey
        reports can be unrealistic and it is almost unheard of for a
        facility to pass a survey without receiving at least one
        deficiency. What you want to look for is the following.
        A: How many deficiencies did they have. B: How severe
        were the deficiencies. C: Was it life threatening.

2   Ask for a tour of the facility so you can see if the residents and
        the facility looks and smells clean.

3   Visit on your own, talk to residents and family members. A
        good time to do this is on the weekend as it's the time that
        most residents family members visit.

4 Ask to meet with the administrator and department heads. This will give you an idea of the type of staffing the facility provides.

5 Contact the activity director and ask him or her to introduce you to the resident council president and or vice president if they have one.

6 Ask the council president or vice about the facility.

7 Request a guest tray for a meal. You may have to pay a small amount for the food, but in most cases this can be done in as little as a two hour notice. You might ask the council president if you could join him or her for a meal. Most facilities provide their main meal for lunch and supper is usually soup and sandwiches.

8 If you can spare as little as one to two hours a month, contact the activity director and ask if you could volunteer to help run a program or attend an outing. You will be surprised how much you will learn about the facility.

9 Ask how many residents they have and how many activity staff are available. There should be no more than forty to forty-five residents for each activity staff employee. If the facility has a sub-acute or Alzheimer's station, add another activity staff person for each of these stations.

#10 Ask to see a copy of the activity calendar and ask the director to explain what the activities are. Some directors list their activities with fancy names and although it may look good at a glance, it could be misleading and be a repeated program with a different title.

#11   Find out how many residents are assigned to each nurse's assistant (C.N.A.). A good rule of thumb is seven or eight residents per care giver.

#12   Find out what your share of the cost will be. This should also cover laundry (if you don't plan to do it yourself) and beauty shop appointments. You can get these answers from the admitting person, accounts receivable person or office manager.

#13   If your doctor has prescribed physical or speech therapy, ask if the facility provides these in-house services.

#14   Ask the social services director what services they provide for the residents and take notes. The minimum service they should provide is to be knowledgeable in financial, Medicare, Medi-Cal, insurance, living wills and the forms needed.

#15   Bear in mind that a nursing home will never replace a person's home. Be it from the care to the food. Staff are taking care of many residents and the doctor's orders have to be followed from food to medication.

CHAPTER 27

DO'S AND DON'TS

If you have exhausted your options and have selected a nursing home for placement the list below will give you recommendations for what you should know.

#1   Make sure when your loved one is admitted that you have a copy of all of their paper work including a copy of the residents rights and the facility directory that lists who to contact if you have a question on a particular matter. If they don't provide this, ask the admitting person to write the department heads names for you.

#2   Give the facility a copy of the living will if there is one. If not the social service department can help you obtain one.

#3   Make sure to give the facility the name and phone numbers of who to contact in case there is an emergency or change in condition that you need be made aware of, the resident's religious belief, pastor's name, name of the mortuary you prefer and any pertinent information that the facility might need to assure your and your loved one's wishes will be carried out.

#4   Most facilities recommend that you bring in personal items such as favorite wall décor and pictures, a favorite chair, television, radio, razor, etc. with the resident's name inscribed on them.   Don't put the room number as residents rooms change at times.

#5   Mark all clothing with a washable marker or paint pens. This us usually done inside the back of the neck for tops and in the waist line for bottoms, the inside of shoes or slippers and on the bottoms of socks.

#6   If you do not plan to do the laundry yourself, do not bring in any clothing that could be ruined by hot water or hot dryer. To protect residents from possible germs, all laundry is done in very hot water and dried in dryers.

#7   If anything is brought in to the resident at a later date, make sure the resident's name is on it. Have the nurse enter it on the resident's inventory list. Lost items will not be replaced if they are not listed on the resident's inventory.

#8   If you are bringing in food items, make sure the nurse knows what food you are bringing. They may need to know what the resident has eaten in case they don't eat all of their meals. Percentages of the meals eaten are charted for weight control or diet restrictions.

#9   If your doctor is unable to visit your family member in the facility, and you have been assigned a doctor, ask when the doctor will be in the facility. Plan to be there or have someone else be at the facility at that time. (Remember my comments regarding some of the nursing home doctors.) The charge nurse at the station where your loved one has been placed can help you with questions regarding the doctors scheduled visits.

#10   Be prepared to attend a resident care plan conference meeting every three months with or without your loved one present. This is your decision, These meetings are to update you on the care the resident is given, how they are responding to their new surroundings, their weight and overall physical condition. Also discussed will be their attendance and participation in activities, if they are socializing and any other pertinent information about the resident. Bear in mind these meetings are usually tried to be kept at no more than twenty minutes. The staff have several other family members to meet with each day so when you attend bring any questions you might have written down to refer to so you won't forget something. This will also speed up the process of the meeting and everything can be covered.

#11   If you work and are not available at the time your care plan conference is scheduled, you can request a conference by telephone. A representative from each department will be available to respond to your questions by conference call.

#12   If there is a particular activity that you want your family member to attend, for instance a religious or musical program, tell the charge nurse on the station that you want the resident up, dressed and taken to the activity. If this is not happening, contact the director of nurses and the activity director.

#13   Visit often, take them for a walk. Attend group programs with them. You will find this is a good way to spend some enjoyable time with them. It is sad but true. Residents who have concerned family or friends visiting often appear to receive more staff attention. Others who have no one to care are often neglected as some care givers don't feel the need to impress an outsider. Most of all, NEVER STOP TELLING THEM YOU LOVE THEM.

CHAPTER 28
WHO TO CONTACT

All facilities consist of several departments that provide care or a service for the residents, but many of them do not have a listing of their department heads and who to contact to retrieve information or get help without going through the process of a lot of red tape to talk the individual in charge of the department where you have a concern or question. The receptionist can give you the names of the administrator and the department heads and the following list should assist you to know what department you need to speak with.

ADMINISTRATOR: Is in charge of the entire facility, they are the person you should speak to if you have not gotten results from the department of where your concern is.

DIRECTOR OF NURSES (D.O.N.): Is in charge of all of the nursing staff. Nursing, health care, cleanliness, personal hygiene or any additional nursing concerns that have been reported to the charge nurse and are not getting resolved should be brought to his or her attention.

QUALITY ASSURANCE NURSE: Is in charge of seeing that quality care is given to the residents and the facility is practicing quality care measures in all departments.

INFECTION CONTROL NURSE: Is in charge of seeing that infection control measures are in affect in a facility.

Some of them also provide orientation for new employees, train the nursing staff and provide in services to inform all staff of pertinent information.

CHARGE NURSES: Are the station supervisor of the other nurses at their stations. If you have a nursing concern you can usually get it resolved by reporting it to the charge nurse at the station where the resident resides.

ADMITTING: Is in charge of all procedures from assigning rooms to the needed paper work for admitting new residents. He or she is usually located in the business office.

ACCOUNTS RECIEVABLE: Is in charge of all monies collected for the facility including a resident's share of cost. They can inform you of what your share of the monthly cost will be.

DIETICIAN: Is in charge of calorie counts, dietary restrictions, meal planning and just about everything that has to do with the residents diets. If you are unhappy with the meals you need to contact either the dietician or the kitchen manager.

SOCIAL SERVICES DEPARTMENT: Is in charge of residents personal matters, scheduling appointments, shopping for clothing if you are unable to do so. They try to resolve disputes between room mates or other residents. They can let you know of room availability if you would like a room change. They also make arrangements for placement in another facility. This can occur when your loved one needs placement in a facility that provides more or less care then they are currently receiving. They can provide you with literature of support groups. They are the department who will contact you to schedule care plan meetings and in turn they are also the department you would contact if you need a conference call in place of attending the care plan meeting.

ACTIVITY DEPARTMENT: Is in charge of all resident activities and recreation, both in house and outings away from the facility. If you have a concern, question or suggestion you should contact the director who is the supervisor of the activity staff.

ENVIROMENTAL SERVICES: Is usually a combination of laundry, housekeeping and the maintenance departments. The maintenance department supervisor usually supervises all three of these departments.

THERAPY DEPARTMENTS: Are in charge of all therapy programs and they all have supervisors. If you have a question regarding therapy you should contact the department supervisor.

CHAPTER 29

OTHER OPTIONS

You have probably heard the term that one has to do a "spend down" down to receive Medical benefits in a nursing home. In the past this was the general consensus. When people were placed in a nursing home they had to spend down their resources to $2500.00 As of January 1, 2002, a person whose spouse is in a nursing home and on Medi-Cal can keep a great deal of their assets, aside from their home and pension plans.

There are many ways to avoid financial hardship. Don't believe there is nothing you can do; there is something you can do to protect you and your spouse's life savings, retirement and home.

The first thing you need to do is to get yourself a qualified senior planning consultant who is knowledgeable on Medicare and Medi-Cal rules.

There are senior citizens services and organizations in the phone book. Before you do anything, contact one of these services and they can direct you to a representative that can assist you in protecting your assets.

However, the best thing you can do to protect your future is to check into these options before you need assistance. Advanced planning will pay off in the end.

CHAPTER 30

CLOSING COMMENTS

In reading about my experiences, I'm sure you realize that my work in nursing homes was not all bad. I had many wonderful, laughable and touching experiences that I wouldn't trade for anything. I have met some wonderful people, have had some excellent staff and volunteers and I have received many blessings.

It is my wish that everyone who reads my book will find it to be interesting, uplifting and amusing. Most of all I hope it will provide informative data and a better understanding of nursing home living and the knowledge of how to research a facility. This gives some control in making a loved ones life "Heaven Or Hell".

ABOUT THE AUTHOR

Joyce Poxon was born in Pekin, Illinois and resided most of her adult life in Crown Point, Indiana relocating to San Diego, California in 1984.

She is the mother of three, five stepchildren and grandmother of eighteen. She began her career in the field of activities in 1980. It was then she realized God had given her a talent to reach out to the elderly and handicapped.

She has been recognized as being one of the best activity directors, trainer and troubleshooter in southern California. Her designed, copyrighted forms and calendar format are used in activity departments of several facilities.

Her recognition includes awards, certificates and references given by Bonita Paradise Management, Baldwin Corporation, Recreation Association, Activity Professionals Association, several geriatric professionals and many individuals.

Printed in the United States
1518600001B/232-477